BE IN BAL

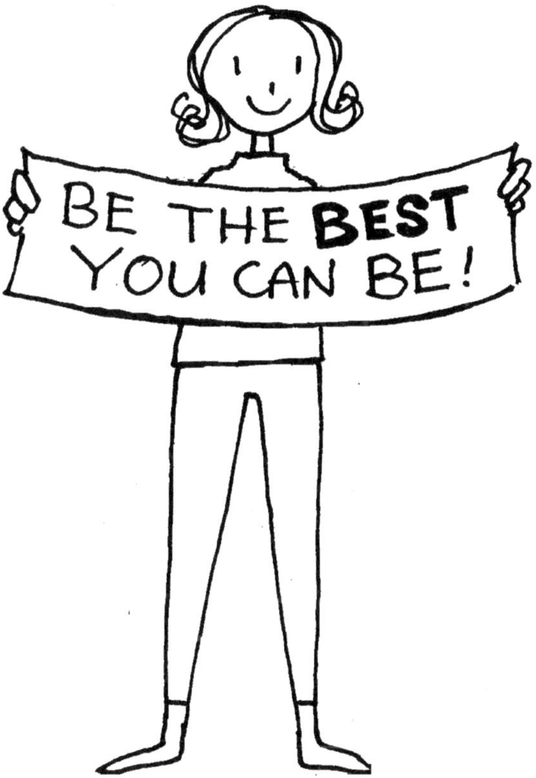

BY ANGELA BRADSHAW MSTAT, DMU, DCR (R)

First published in 2014 Balloon View Ltd, Kent, TN26 2DD

ISBN: 978-1-907798-34-4

Printed and bound in Great Britain by CPI Group (UK) Ltd, Croydon, CR0 4YY

INTRODUCTION

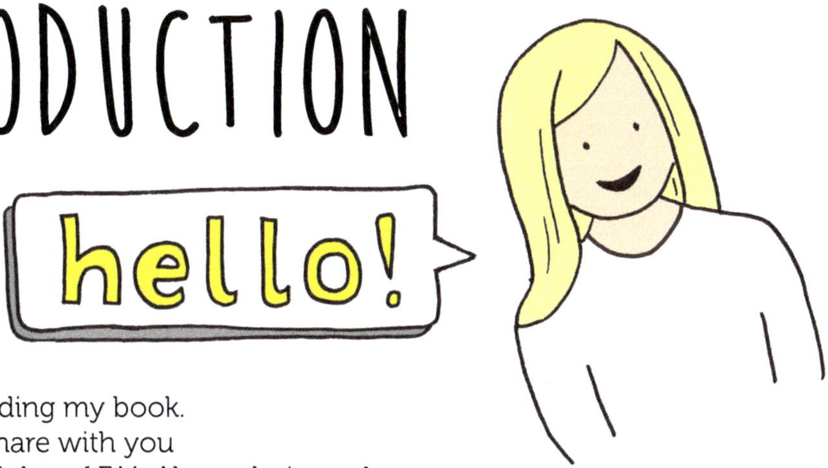

Thank you for reading my book.
I'm delighted to share with you
some of the principles of F.M. Alexander's work.

This is a simple introduction to the Alexander Technique (AT), and is NOT a substitute for a hands-on lesson with a qualified teacher. The 'real deal' is a unique experience, which is difficult to articulate.

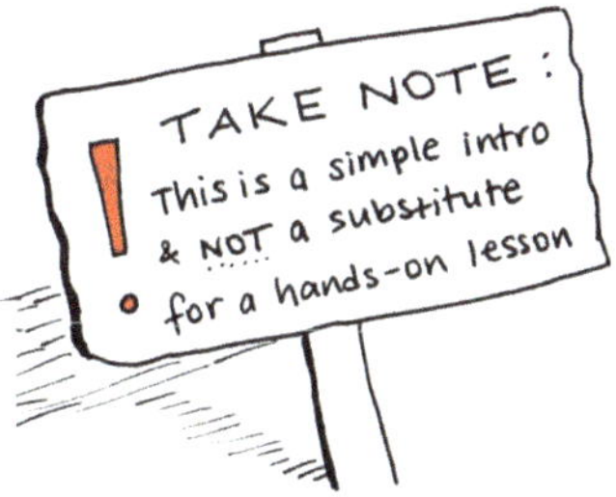

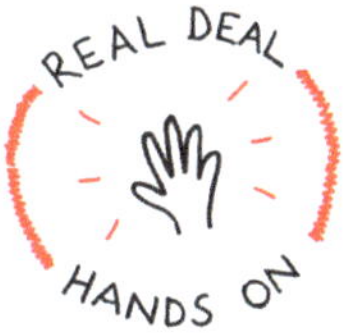

Aldous Huxley described his experience of lessons with F.M. Alexander as akin to describing the colour red to a blind person who had never had the gift of sight.

Everyone's experience of AT is unique to the individual to whom it is tailored.

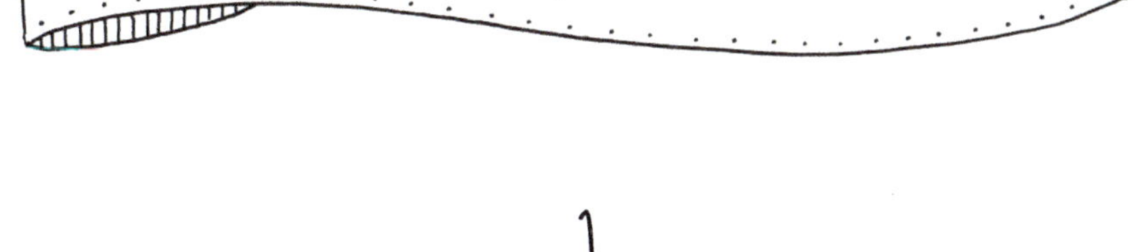

But we are all humans sharing this planet at the same time and we do have many common problems. This book was borne out of my personal wish to bring the work of F.M. Alexander into the mainstream in an accessible way.

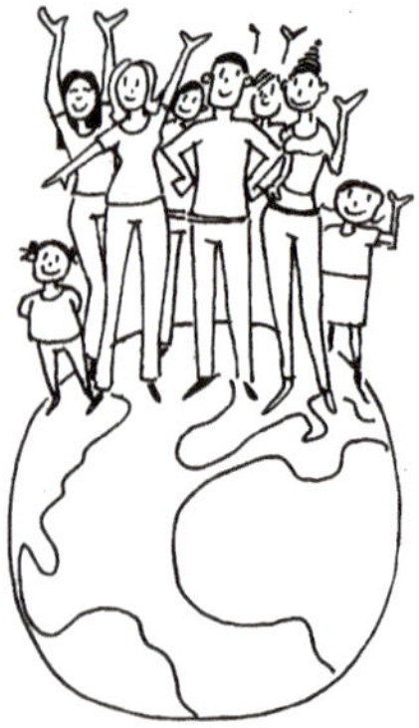

The work is simple, yet takes commitment to practise. After all, we are up against our personal habits!

AND simple does not always mean easy!

But if you have the will and the wish to learn, it pays **HUGE** dividends to your health, wellbeing, sensory awareness, balance, co-ordination, posture, energy levels, thinking skills, mindfulness, spatial awareness, performance, breathing, handling anxiety, handling stress ... the list goes on.

Who is this book for?

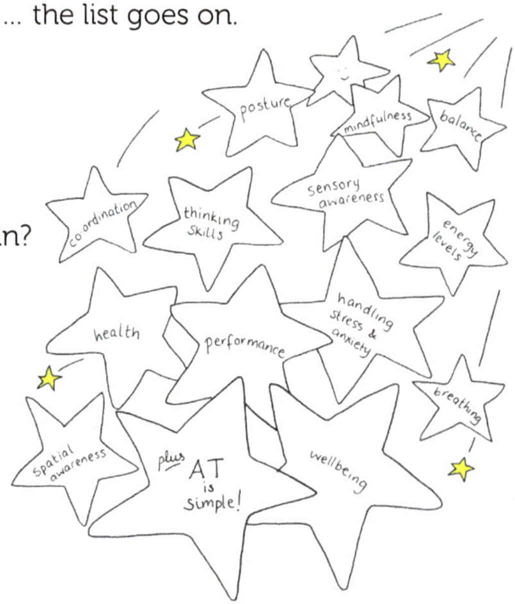

Do you

- have back/shoulder/neck pain?
- have RSI issues?
- have posture concerns?
- suffer from anxiety?
- suffer from stress?
- struggle with confidence?

Are you

- a professional person?
- a musician?
- a cyclist?
- a runner?
- an athlete?
- an actor?
- pregnant?
- wanting to improve yourself?

Then read on ... the Alexander Technique can help **YOU** to **BE IN BALANCE**...it's the **BEST** that you can be

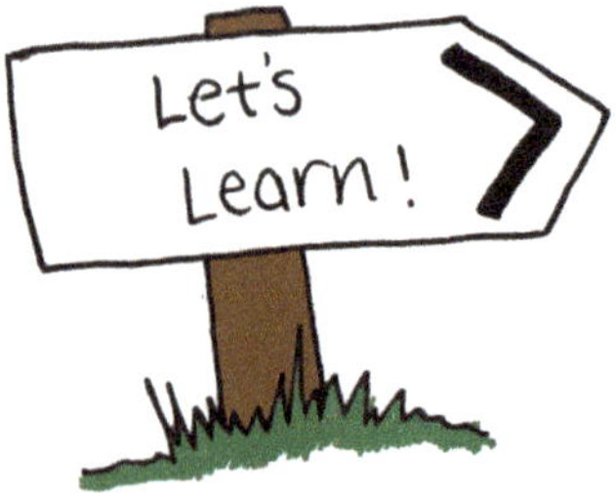

ABOUT THE AUTHOR

Angela Bradshaw originally trained as a sonographer and radiographer, and enjoyed some years in this profession.

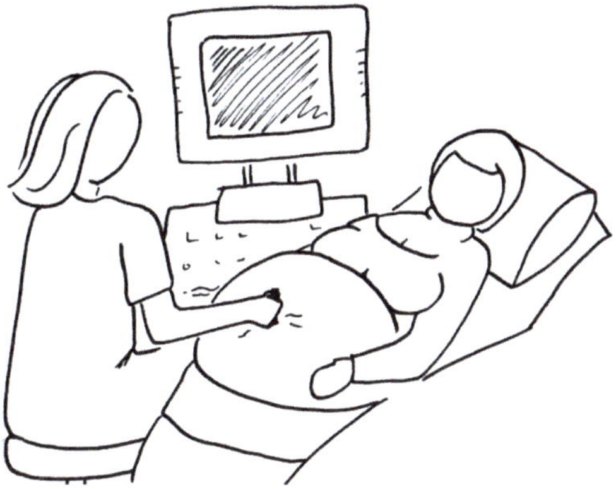

However, a repetitive strain injury curtailed this career, and in seeking help for this she discovered the Alexander Technique.

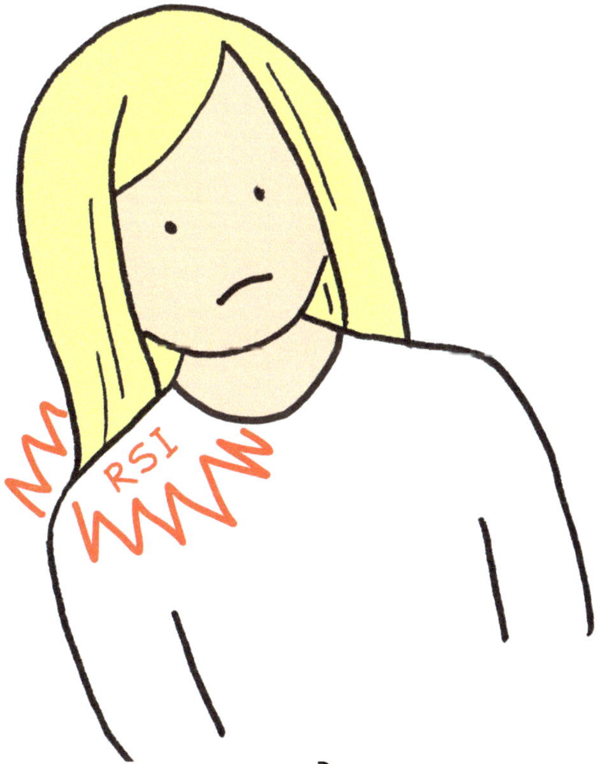

When she realised what a profound effect the technique could have on this type of injury, and also the broad scope of its applications, she decided to become a teacher herself. She now works with individuals and groups, using the Alexander Technique to help them learn how to use their bodies well.

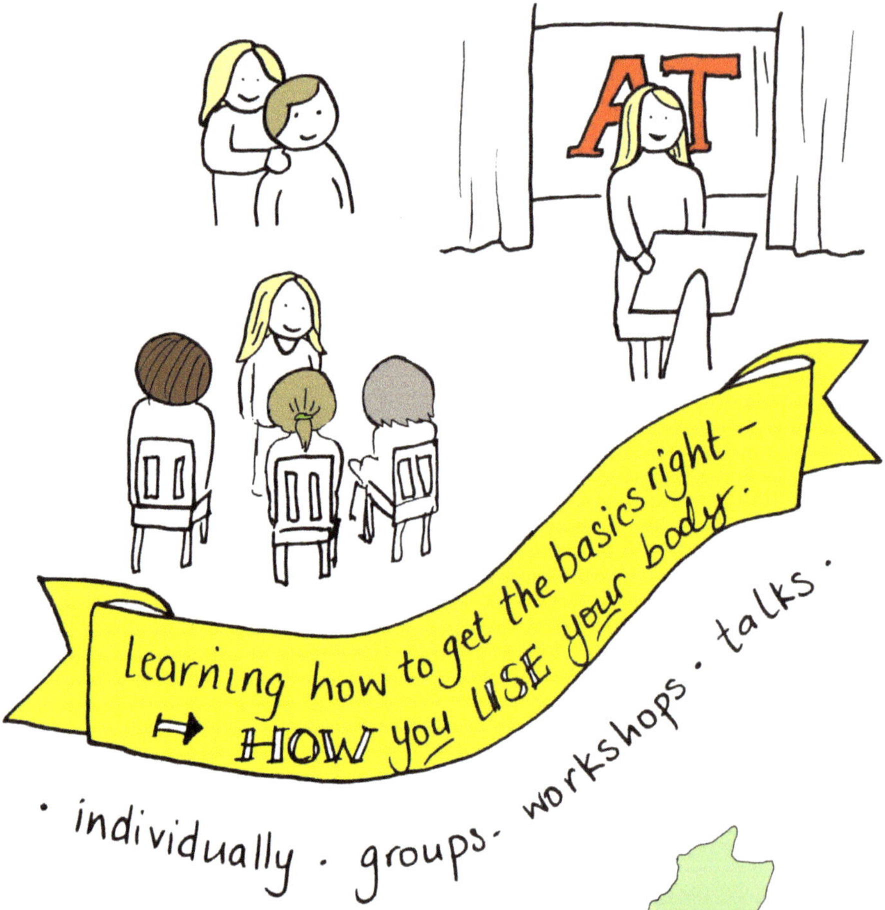
AT
learning how to get the basics right –
→ HOW you USE your body.
· individually · groups · workshops · talks ·

Angela lives with her husband, Keith, and their two daughters, Heather and Grace, in Woking, Surrey.

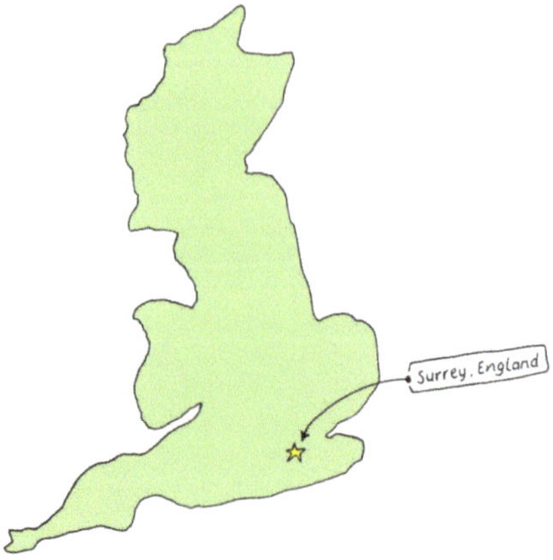

WHO WAS F.M. ALEXANDER?

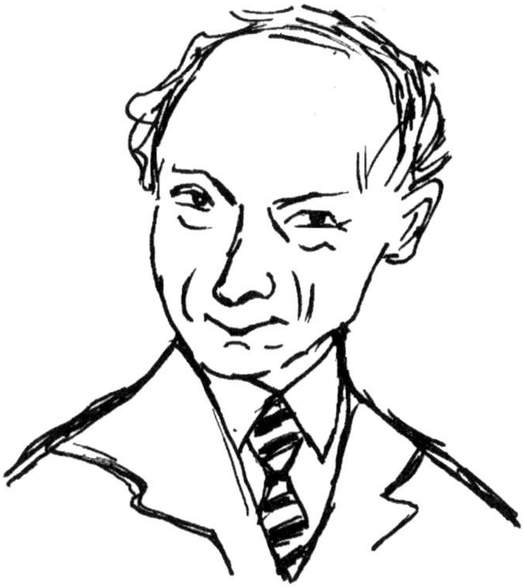

Frederick Matthias Alexander was a man ahead of his time. As a young Shakespearean actor in the 1890s, he had a problem that threatened to end his promising career. His voice would become increasingly hoarse during performances until he was barely audible. He consulted doctors about it, but no underlying medical cause or disease could be found. Rest would restore his voice, but another performance would soon render it gone again!

He reasoned that it was something he was doing himself to cause this strain on his vocal organs. His only option was self-help. Using mirrors, he observed his way of speaking and thus the work was begun.

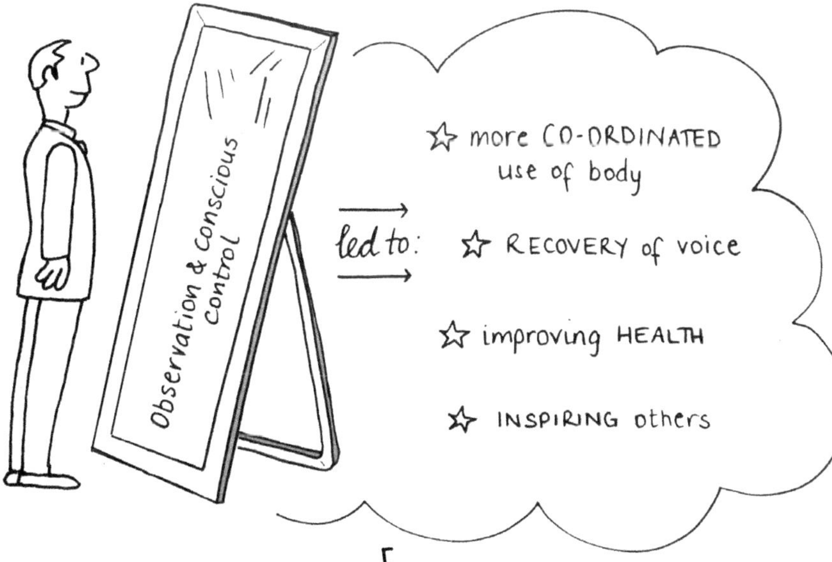

Over a period of several years he realised that the poor coordination of his whole being had led to this original 'problem'. Conscious control of his actions led to a more coordinated use of himself, and he recovered his voice and improved his own health. The development of his Technique began when other people came to him for help with issues of their own.

The medical profession referred patients to him, actors flocked to him and the Technique became his main occupation. He subsequently came to London where he taught the Technique until his death in 1955.

There are 2,500 Alexander Technique teachers worldwide as I write in 2013.

WHO USES THE ALEXANDER TECHNIQUE?

WRITERS

George Bernard Shaw
Aldous Huxley
Roald Dahl

MUSICIANS

Lulu
Madonna
Michael Ball
Paul McCartney

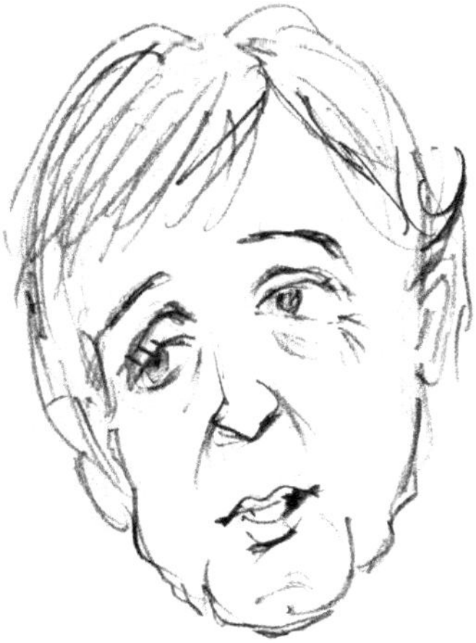

ACTORS

Alan Cummings
Judi Dench
Maggie Smith
Hilary Swank
Hugh Jackman
Jennifer Saunders
Jeremy Irons
Joanna Lumley
John Cleese
Julie Andrews
Juliet Stevenson
Kevin Kline
Lenny Henry
Patrick Stewart
Paul Newman
Robin Williams
Sheila Hancock
Michael Caine
Terence Stamp
William Hurt
Joanne Woodward
Alec McCowan

SPORTS PEOPLE

Daley Thompson
John McEnroe
Greg Chappell
Linford Christie
Howard Payne (Commonwealth record hammer thrower)
Valerie Thompson-Williams (rowing masters gold medallist)

OTHERS

Joan Bakewell
Lisa Snowdon
Andrew Logan (Sculptor)

SOME ALEXANDER TECHNIQUE 'CELEBRITIES'

Judi Dench

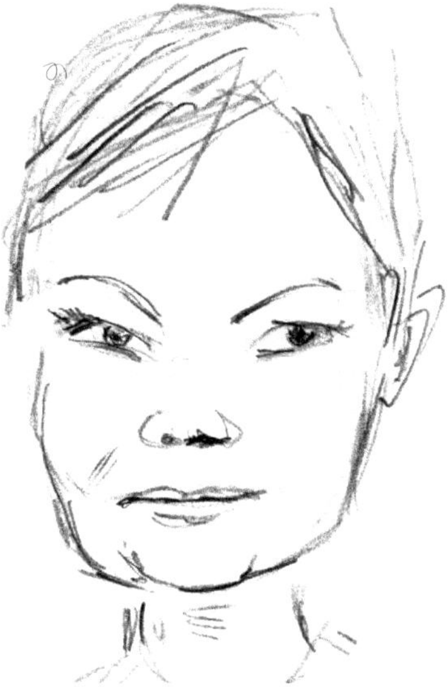

Joanna Lumley

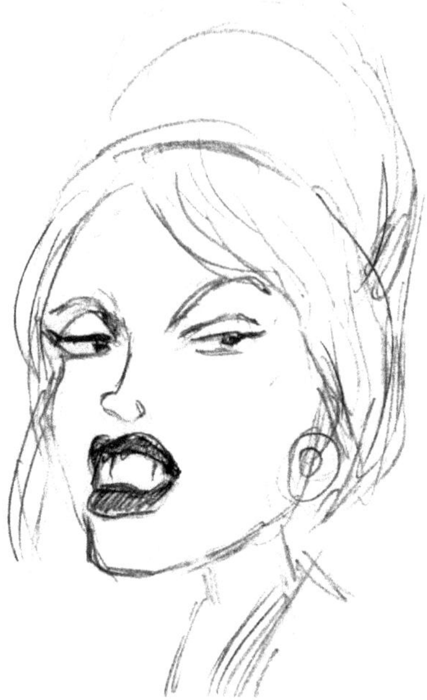

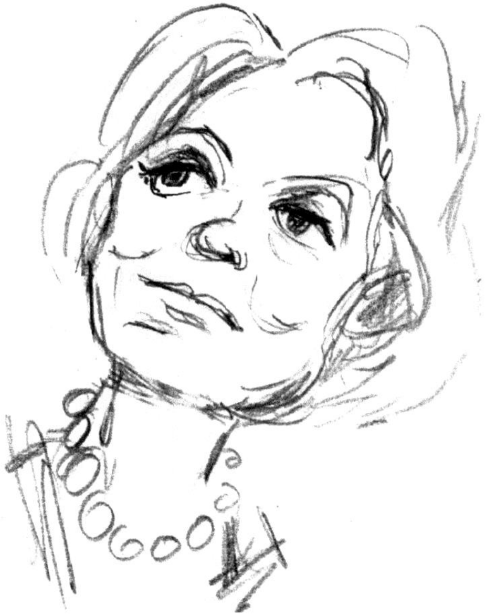

Maggie Smith

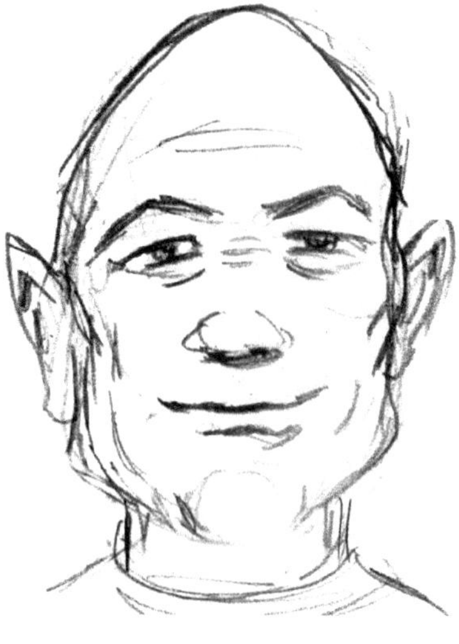

Patrick Stewart

Book Reviews

"While relaxing on the south coast, a few days before reading the draft of Angela Bradshaw's Be In Balance, I received an urgent message, which necessitated my making an international call on my mobile phone. A virtually non-existent signal, a boisterous wind, the need to conduct a critical negotiation with an excited respondent whose broken English was delivered with machine-gun rapidity…What could possibly go wrong?

If only I'd already had the benefit of reading Angela's book, which introduces the Alexander Technique to the uninitiated, I would have handled the situation better. I could have approached the call the Alexander way (yes, as Angela points out, the Technique can be applied to every aspect of everyday life, even telephone behaviour). As it was, in the heat of the moment I forgot what very little I already knew of the Alexander Technique. Shouting into that mobile phone, worrying about the content of the conversation, not hearing and not being heard, I tensed up: shoulders high, breathing shallow, knees locked rather than (as Angela puts it) 'on the latch' – it was a classic recipe for postural disaster. My distressed right-side gluteus minimus muscle, which had given me long-term problems but was on the mend, relapsed into painful spasm.

Can such tension, and its unfortunate and sometimes painful consequences, really be avoided? In Be In Balance, Angela Bradshaw sets out to show that it can. For the Alexander follower, the demands of civilisation, and of today's hectic life in particular, have made us forget or abandon the natural, relaxed movements and postures of childhood. Angela, herself a former sufferer from a repetitive strain injury, has dedicated herself to reminding us how the body naturally wants to be, and how the Alexander Technique can help us to achieve this. Be In Balance is not a substitute for lessons with a 'hands-on' teacher, but it is a welcome, no-nonsense introduction to the Technique, made with wit, obvious passion and infectious enthusiasm, which should encourage its readers to progress to the next stage of 'being in balance'."

Mike Hewitt MSc –
Medical Copy Writer

"Read the book and then have lessons, or have lessons then read the book – either way, you can't go wrong. I had my first series of lessons 30 years ago and still have monthly top-ups."

Norman Chancer – Actor

"This book is absolutely brilliant. It is very reader-friendly, fluent and has a great flow. I love the use of different text, humour and expressions, as well as the visual demonstrations, which are great all the way through."

Lisa Craig – Physiotherapist

"Angela has written a wonderfully practical handbook that explains the Alexander Technique in very down-to-earth terms and makes its wisdom and techniques accessible to all. This brilliant book heightens body awareness and highlights simple postural changes that can be integrated into all aspects of daily life. I will certainly recommend this excellent, easy to follow guide to all my patients."

Jennifer Harper-Deacon, Registered Naturopathic Physician, author, Health Journalist of the Year 2008 and former 'What's the Alternative?' columnist, The Sunday Times

"This refreshingly written short book is easy to follow and entertaining and I found myself swept along with Angela's enthusiasm for this new way of 'being'.

While reading the book, I immediately had to try the techniques described and it just all seemed to make sense. What a refreshing change from being told to 'keep your shoulders back and hold your stomach in'!

I was familiar with the Technique before reading this book, but Angela opened my eyes to the many beneficial effects that it could potentially bring, for example, improving the musician's performance on his instrument or helping the public speaker.

This is an easy read, which could have a huge impact and be potentially life changing for many people."

Brenda Walton – Lead Sonographer

"An excellent, clear book that has inspired me to consider my own posture and beliefs about everything in my life, from how I sit at my desk to putting myself first. There are some great metaphors to illustrate points and the book is written at such a level that you can follow it easily. Inspiring, positive and potentially life changing!"

Gill Harrison – Ultrasound Programme Director.

CHAPTER ONE

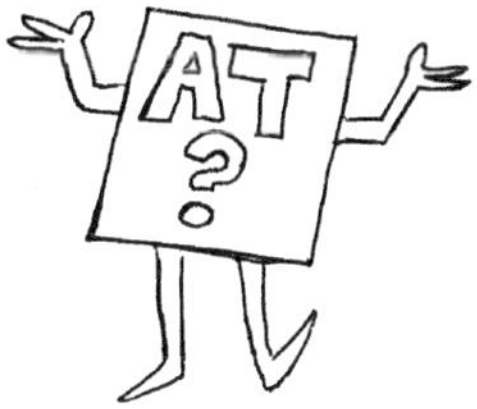

WHAT IS THE ALEXANDER TECHNIQUE?

The Alexander Technique is a self-help solution for the common problem of poor posture and the associated loss of balance and mal-co-ordination that comes with it. Certified registered teachers of the Alexander Technique use hands-on guidance to help teach people to recover their natural posture by learning **HOW** to use their body well.

You see, there is a choice in **HOW** to use your body. The good news is that you've already experienced using your body well before! When we are babies and young toddlers, we have effortless use of our bodies. Movement is free and easy because we aren't interfering with our inherent poise and balance.

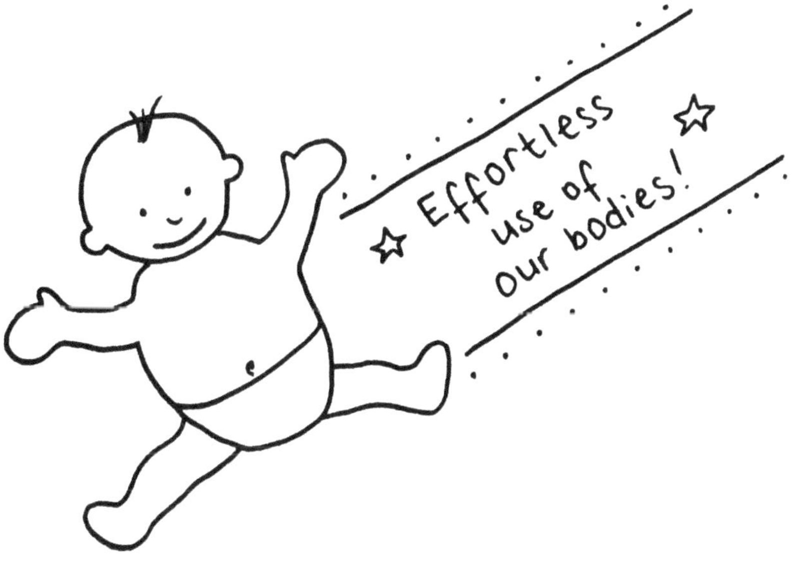

So when we learn **HOW** to use our body well again, it's a huge relief.
That was great news to me when I discovered the work of F.M. Alexander.

I knew a lot about anatomy, being a radiographer and sonographer, yet I wasn't applying that knowledge to myself. I certainly wasn't using my body well. For many years I had been told I had poor posture, and I had wrongly assumed that it was inherited, thanks to a poor gene pool combination!

Why is posture important?

Posture directly affects how well you function. It has a significant effect on your health and wellbeing. Yet we know very little about how we co-ordinate ourselves. No one teaches us. We learn by ourselves through trial and error as healthy babies and toddlers.

Nature helps us in the process and at that young age we are still 'using' our bodies relatively well.

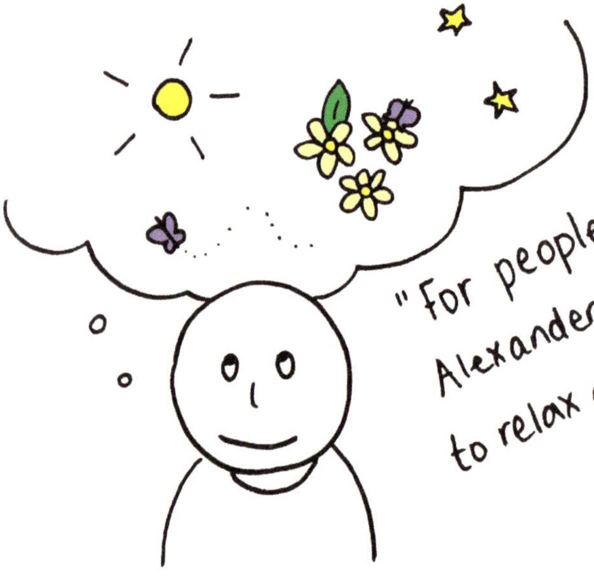

"For people who live in their heads, Alexander Technique is a GREAT way to relax and connect with your body."

– TRUDY DELAMERE, BUSINESS COACH

Why do we go wrong?

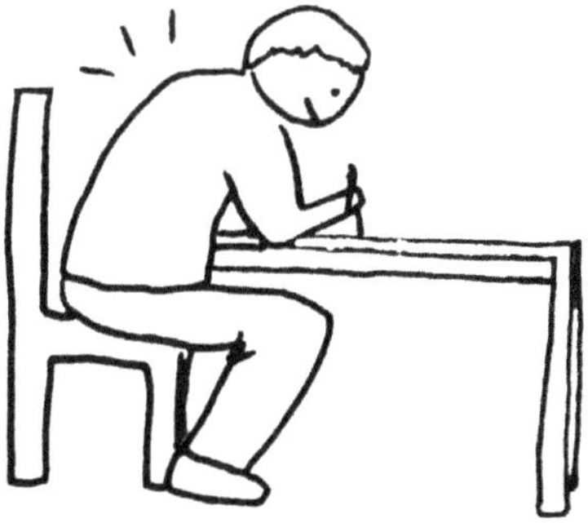

For a myriad of reasons, we begin to adopt unhelpful habits of movement as we get older. We go to school and sit for long periods of time hunched over desks on chairs that aren't supportive.

We are less physically active than ever before. Babies are carried about in curved car seats, hardly ever getting an opportunity to lengthen their little spines. Silver Cross prams are a thing of the past, replaced by lightweight buggies – very convenient for transporting little people around, but unhelpful in terms of their healthy physical development. Nappies can interfere with a toddler's gait when learning to walk. And shoes can restrict feet and encourage toddlers to learn to bear weight unnaturally.

Our children now get less physical exercise than ever before, and this problem is further compounded by the technology prevalent in modern society.

Television, computers, smart phones, games consoles...
they all encourage a sedentary lifestyle.

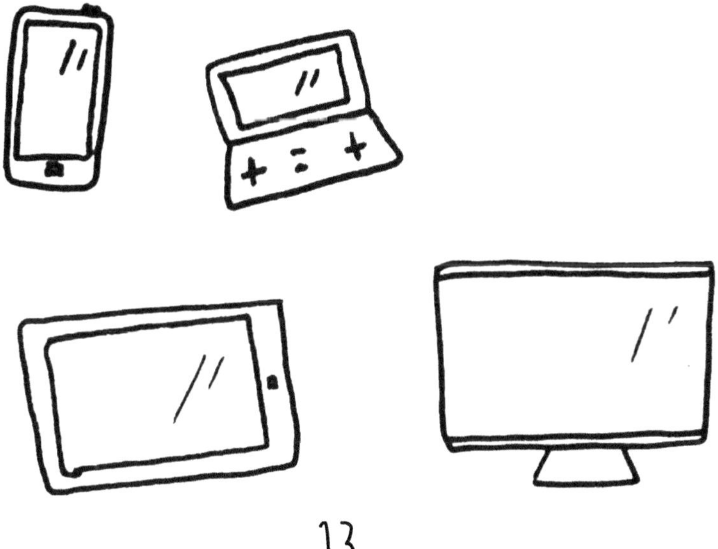

Issues of safety mean we don't encourage our children to roam outdoors and amuse themselves, as we were encouraged to do in our youth, and that's not so long ago!

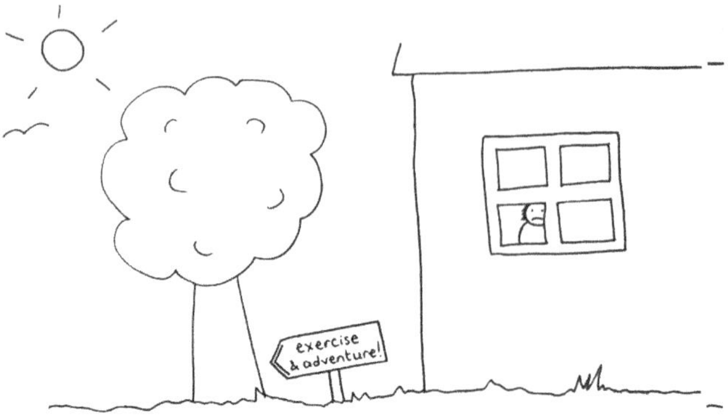

Schools keep children inside at break times if it's raining for health and safety reasons, further diminishing opportunities for free physical play.

We also might mimic the movements, gait and postural habits of our parents and adopt them as 'normal'. We are very influenced by our lifestyles, our peers, our parents, the people who surround us and the environment we live in, not to mention the quality of our diet, and whether we get enough rest and physical exercise.

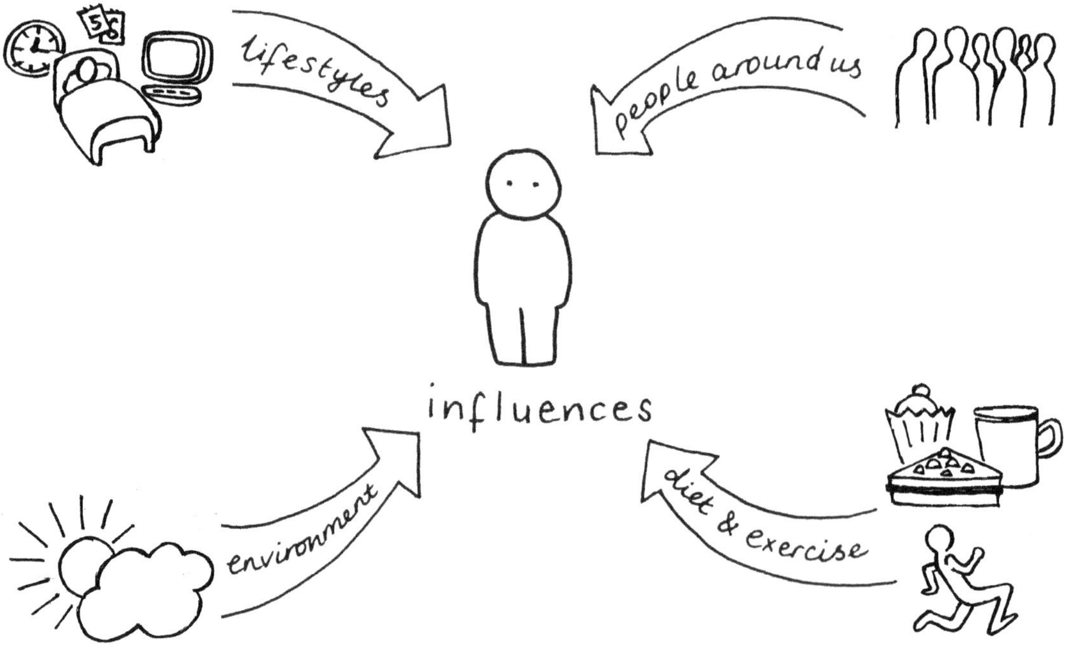

CHAPTER TWO

HOW CAN THE ALEXANDER TECHNIQUE HELP ME?

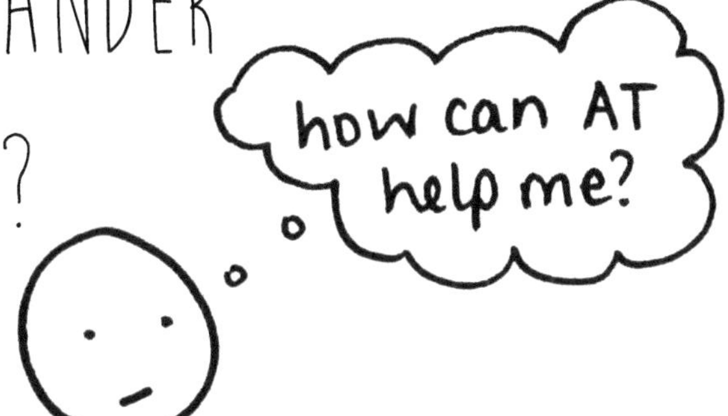

You might well be wondering ...

In truth it can help **EVERYONE** and **ANYONE** who is open and willing to learn! There's always room for improvement in the way we use our bodies. This work makes us conscious of **HOW** we use our body, **HOW** we think, **HOW** we move and **HOW** we balance.

It's...

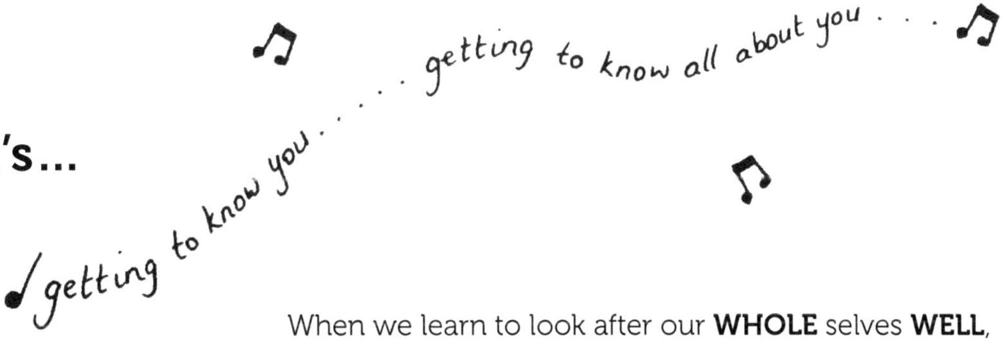

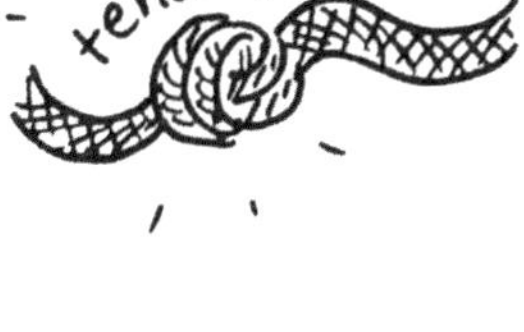

When we learn to look after our **WHOLE** selves **WELL**, we become more responsible for ourselves. We learn how to respond appropriately to our circumstances. We can release a lot of physical tension, which frees up a huge amount of our energy. We learn to be economical with effort and efficient with our energy. Imagine that! Doesn't that sound like a great state to be in?

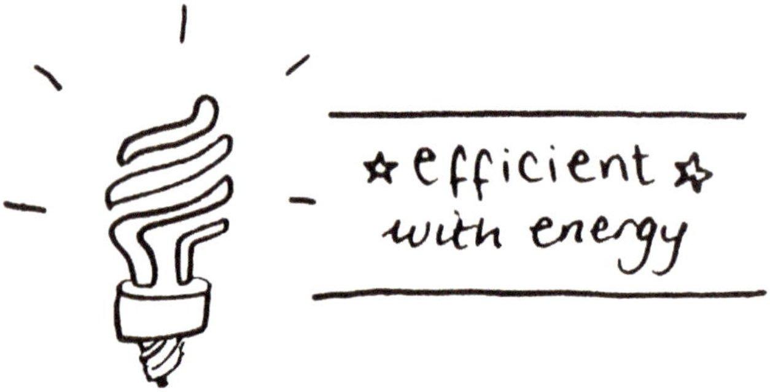

It can be yours – with practice you can access this free and easy natural state more and more often.

The Alexander Technique truly is self-help that you can apply to yourself whenever you want to. Even in challenging circumstances it's still available like a pocket friend patiently waiting until you are ready to use it.

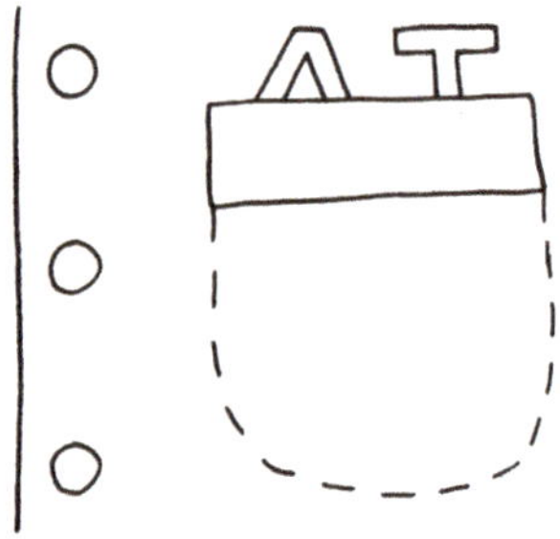

"AT helped me realise that I do have a connection with my body and it's not just a vehicle that moves me around. The way we move our body is so important and it needs to be treated with respect. I found AT has been a wonderful tool that works well with my yoga practice. I felt that my yoga was just the connection that was needed but, after experiencing some AT sessions, I was amazed at the new connections I had made with my body's movement. AT is a skill that everyone needs, however connected they think they are."

Sarah Caswell – Kundalini Yoga Teacher

Q Are you ready?

YES Show me how!

First let's have a whistle-stop anatomy tour so at least you understand **WHAT'S WHERE** in **YOU**.

You see, we think we know ... but it really does no harm to take another look and **REALLY** find out how it all works ...

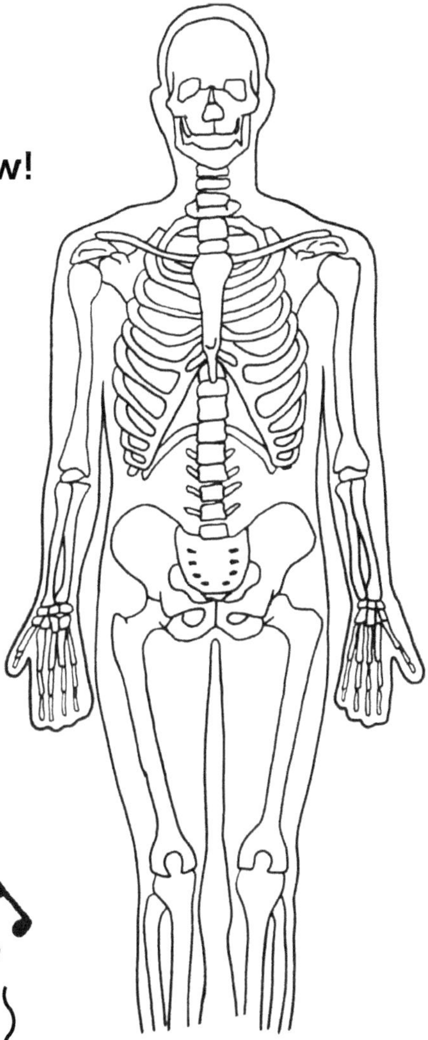

DEM BONES

DEM BONES, DEM BONES

The toe bone connects to the ... **FOOT** bone.
The foot bone connects to the ... **ANKLE** bone ...

And so on

That was one of my favourite songs at school!

I like to start with ...

FEET

Did you know that in nature, when we're standing or sitting, **FULL FOOT** contact with the ground means equal contact between these three points and the floor?

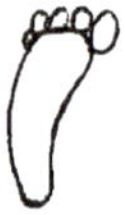

the base of the big toe

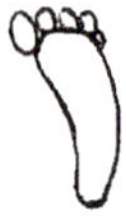

the base of the little toe

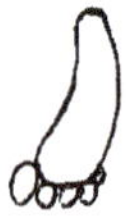

AND the heel

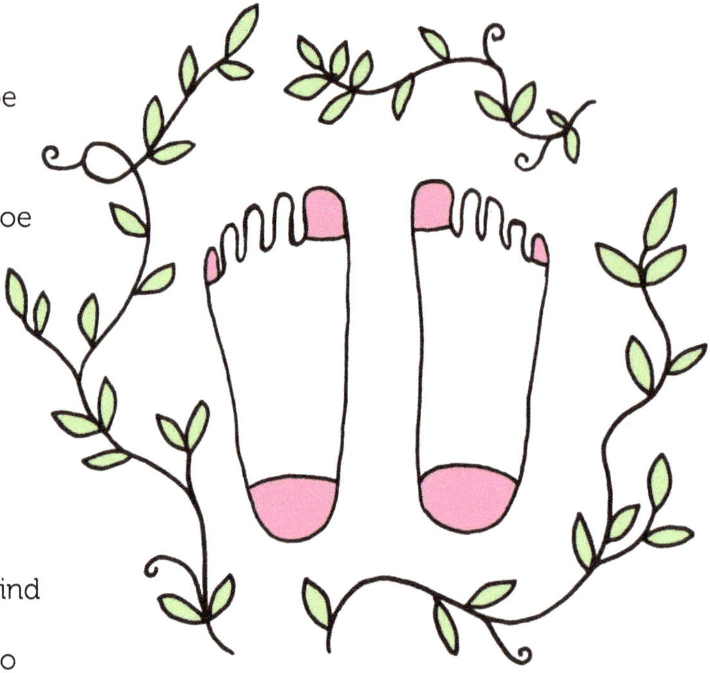

Check in with yourself and find out what your preference is. We usually favour one or two of those points of contact.

I am **YET** to find a client who, when I begin work with them, actually stands in perfect balance, evenly distributing their body weight between both feet and sharing it across all three points of contact equally.

So, you're now meeting some of **YOUR** own personal habits! Interesting isn't it? And we've only just begun!

Next stop ... ANKLES

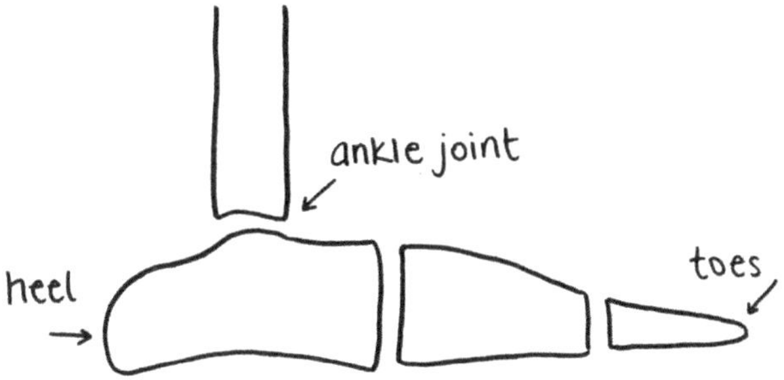

Incidentally, ankles are a long way in front of the heels!

Feel your ankle bones, now feel the back of your heel. Feel how wide it is, too. Shocked? So was I! This was despite my many years as a radiographer. I had been X-raying ankles in A&E departments and orthopaedic clinics, so intellectually I knew very well the anatomy of an ankle joint **IN OTHER PEOPLE!** In myself, however, I had incorrectly bodymapped my ankle something more like this:

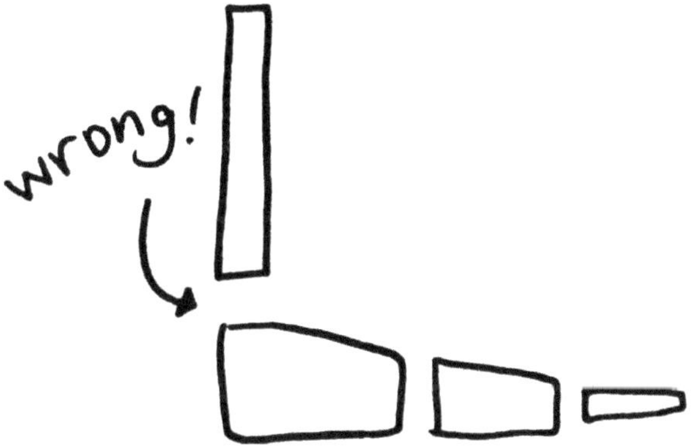

You catch my drift? In my mind I was sending messages to an ankle joint further down and further back than it **ACTUALLY** was.

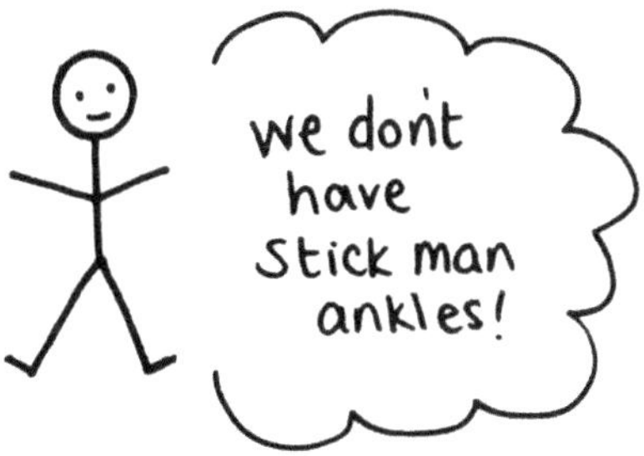

Isn't it amazing what a small amount of information with a bit of attention can deliver? Life changing freedom in my ankles is now mine – and can be yours too!

LOWER LEG...
We have two bones in the lower leg:

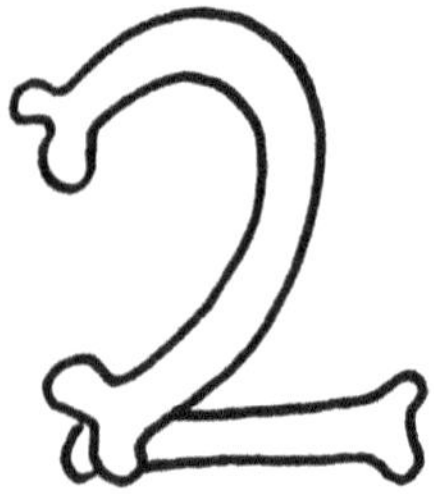

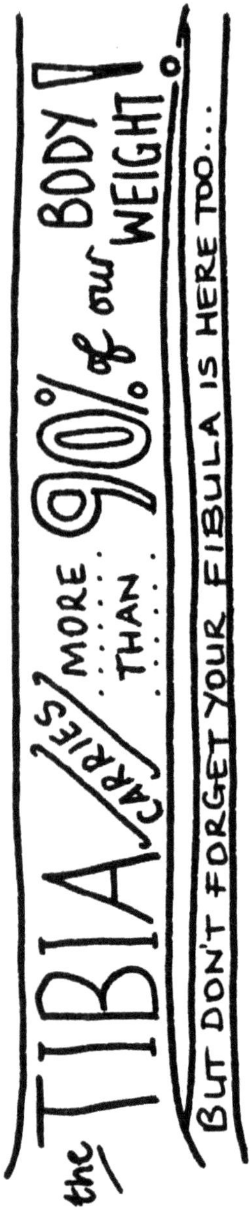

We're all very familiar with the shin bone. We can feel it. Go on, have a prod. Yes, that one! You may have previously found your shin bone painfully when bumping into furniture in the dark!

The **TIBIA** (shin bone) is responsible for taking a lot of our body weight when we're standing (approximately 90-95%).

Now, it also has a quiet friend in the lower leg: the **FIBULA**. This bone we're not so familiar with. It's covered in muscle; we can't feel most of it. We can only feel the fibula on the outer edge of the ankle joint. It plays an important role in ankle mobility **AND** it does play a small role in weight bearing (approximately 5-10%, depending on which medical textbook you're reading!) when we're standing. Yet many of us don't include it in our thinking.

So when you stand or sit, **CONSIDER YOUR FIBULA**; think around the outer edge of your calf and see what happens. Another discovery - and a very enlivening process!

KNEE JOINT

Notice your kneecap; give that a feel. Now let your kneecap fall away from your hip. You just experienced a thigh lengthening moment! Bliss!

Knee-caps sit IN **FRONT** of the knee joint. They are actually **NOTHING** to do with the action of bending the knee. Yet many of us believe it is necessary to pull up the knee-cap in order to bend the knee.

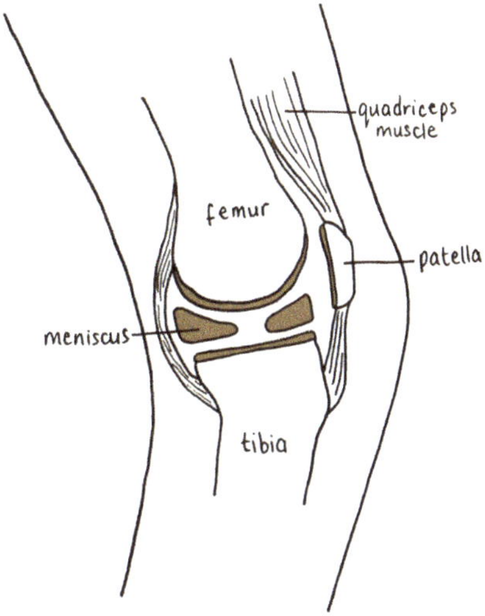

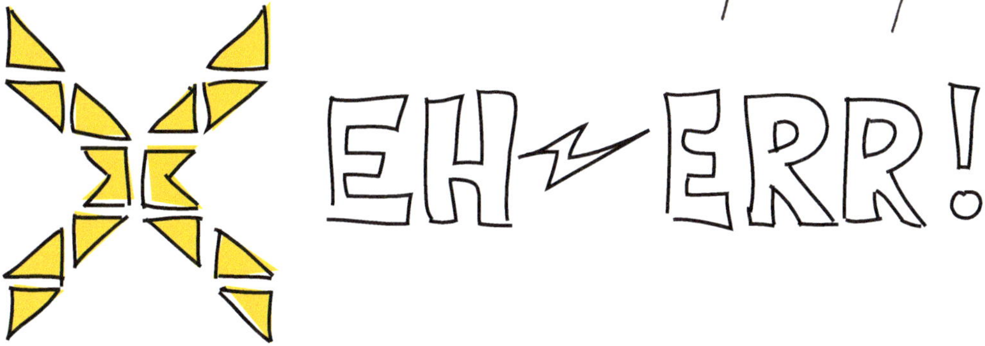

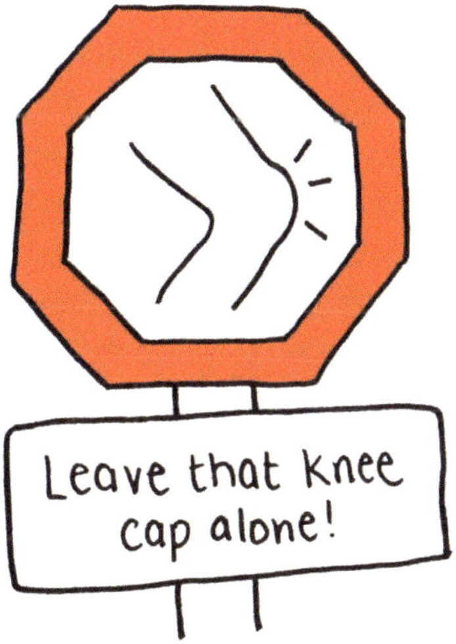

You're now learning to leave the kneecap alone!

Think of the knee joint as bending from the back of the joint through to the front. Remember your shin bone (tibia) is wide – give it due space in your thinking.

Yes, that's right, knees should be **SOFT** and 'on the latch', available for movement – **NOT LOCKED**!

THIGH BONE

The femur connects hip to knee.

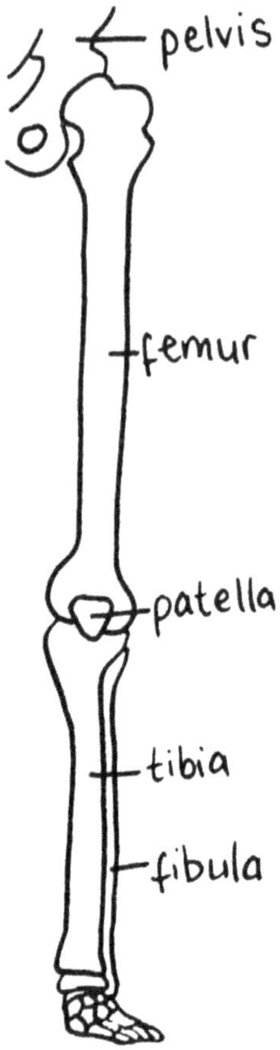

HIP JOINT

Where are the hips?

Feel the crests of your pelvis.

Now find the bony protrusion on the front aspect of your pelvis. A third of the way between this bony protrusion (known as the ASIS – Anterior Superior Iliac Spine) and the pubic bone, almost in the knicker line, is the location of the **HIP JOINT**.

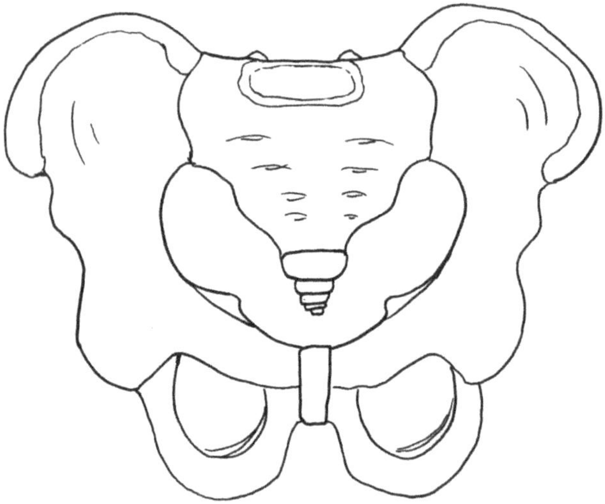

Yes, it's that low down. The English language doesn't help us in our body mapping. 'Hips' refers to a variety of anatomical places and includes hip joints and iliac crests, which are geographically far apart from each other. Confusion can easily arise from this and again messages can be sent to the wrong address!

Ask the muscles around the head of the femur to lengthen and release the leg away from the pelvis.

We all tend to **HOLD** our limbs closely to our torso.

What we want, however, is to maximise the available space in the joints so our movements are **FREER**.

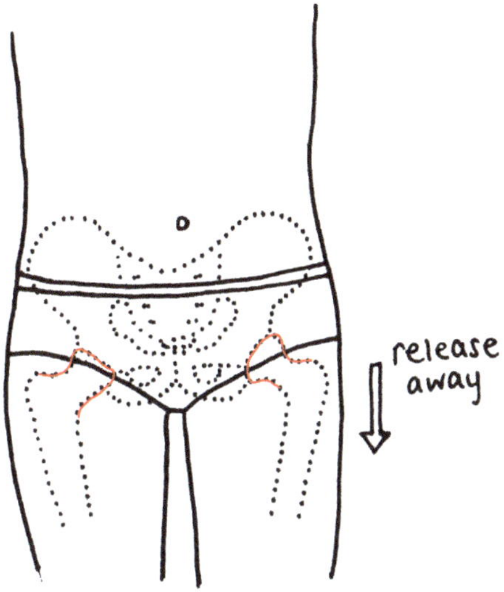

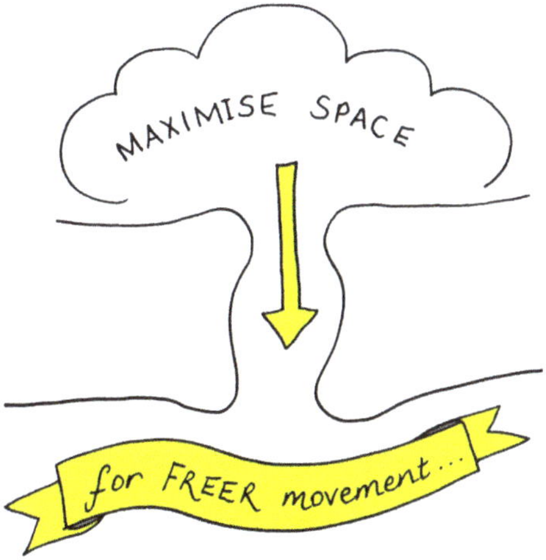

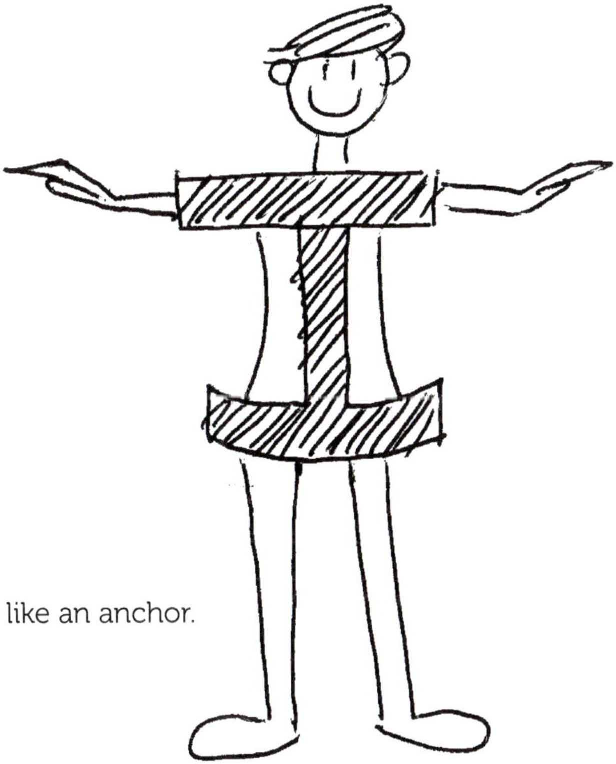

PELVIS

Let your pelvis hang from your head like an anchor.

Where is my SPINE?

Remember that old-fashioned saying "Put your back into it!" My gran used to say that to me all the time – obviously I wasn't doing it very often!

So where is your spine? OK, feel the bony protrusion on the outer edge of the thigh just a short distance away from your hip joint. Your tail bone (coccyx) is at this level.

This is the lower end of your spine.

Notice the spine is **CURVED** and not **STRAIGHT**. Sometimes we have a misconception that we need to straighten out our spines.

Curves are good! But of course only the curves that are appropriate and in the natural direction.

The lumbar spine curves forwards away from the coccyx; the thoracic spine curves backwards in relation to the lumbar spine; and the cervical spine has two natural curves. Gray's Anatomy is a great medical anatomy textbook if you want detail. For the purposes of this book, I'm deliberately only giving a simple overview.

The top of the spine is all the way up here ... put your fingers in your ears. The top of the spine is this high up, between the ears and behind the eyes. This is a revelation to many people!

This joint, the atlanto-occipital joint, is the **MOST IMPORTANT JOINT** in us all.

A LONG – spine – is a STRONG spine

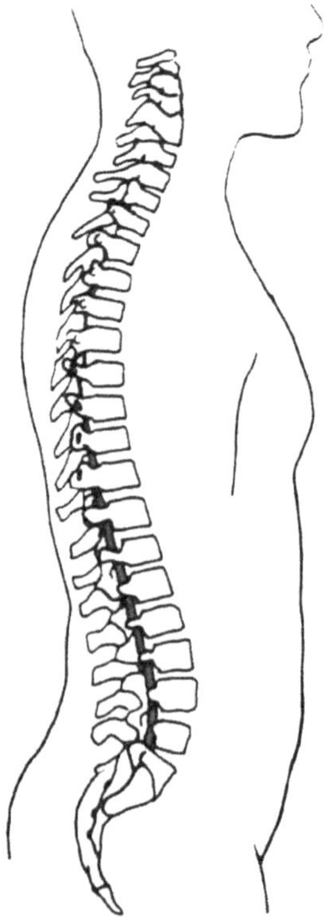

Alexander's unique discovery was this: the arrangement of the head, neck and back is of the upmost importance. It determines how well co-ordinated we are in movement. He called it the **PRIMARY CONTROL**.

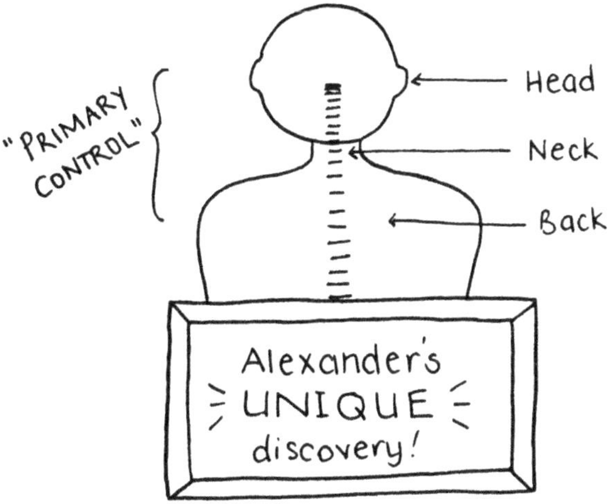

HEAD

The adult head weighs approximately 4.5 kilos.
Find something of a similar weight – a large bag of potatoes, a gym weight, a couple of bags of sugar, a cat. Yes you'll notice how **HEAVY** it is!

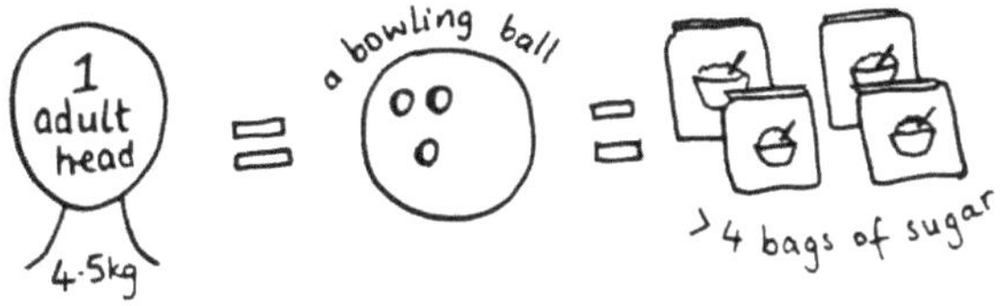

You want to **WEAR YOUR HEAD WELL**.

Why? So that its weight is distributed down the vertebral bodies of the spine as nature intended.

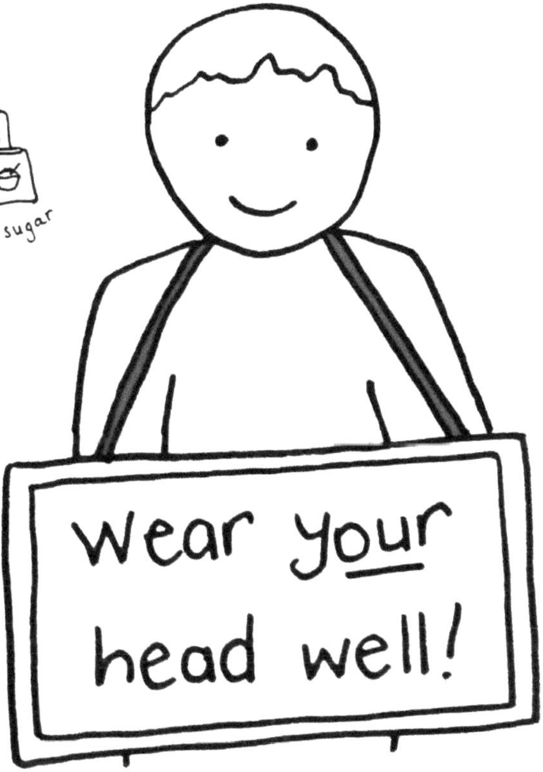

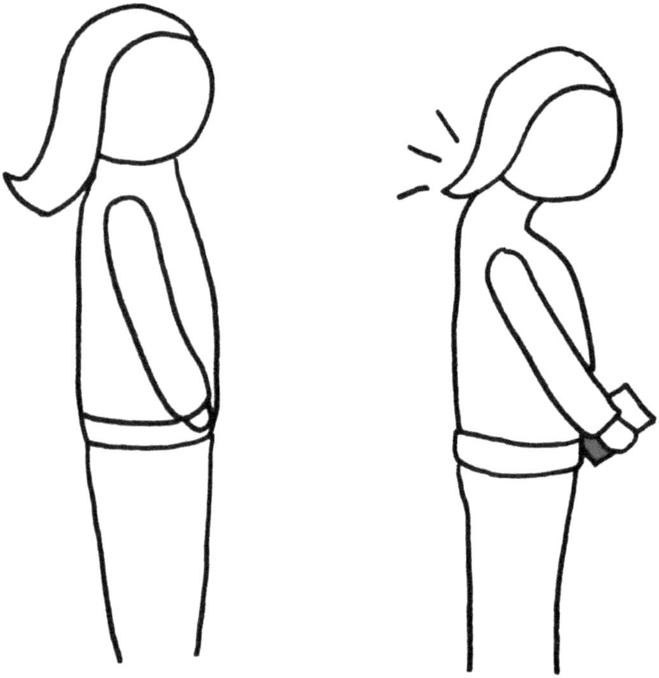

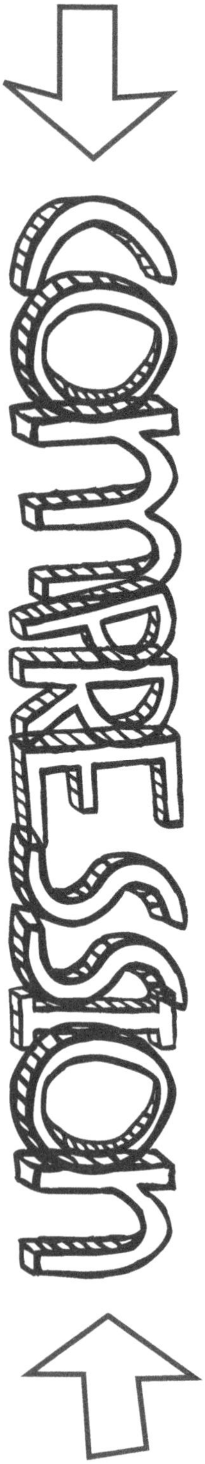

Many of us pull our heads back and down unconsciously. This distributes the head weight down the back of the spine along the spinous processes (not what nature intended, apart from an urgent issue of survival – more on that later).

The action of pulling the head back and down also compresses the spinal column.

We maintain this state for unnaturally **LONG** periods of time in our busy, modern, stressful lives.

So allow your head to rebalance now. Try this: put your fingers in your ears again, briefly. This is the fulcrum of motion, the point where your head meets your spine, the most important joint, the atlanto-occipital joint.

Most of the weight of the head is in front of the spine when we aren't interfering with its natural balance. Added to that is the weight of the jaw.

Send your eyes to look at the ground below you. Breathe; let your tummy out. Now allow gravity to act on your head, pulling it forwards and away from the top of the spine.

Send your eyes up to look straight ahead. Your head is now closer to a more natural alignment.

It may well 'feel' wrong as it's against your habit. But we can't trust feelings as we have faulty sensory awareness.

Experiment with nodding your head gently, keeping the top (atlanto-occipital) joint free and available.

Your head can freely balance on the top of your spine; it's done it before and it can do so again when **YOU** allow it!

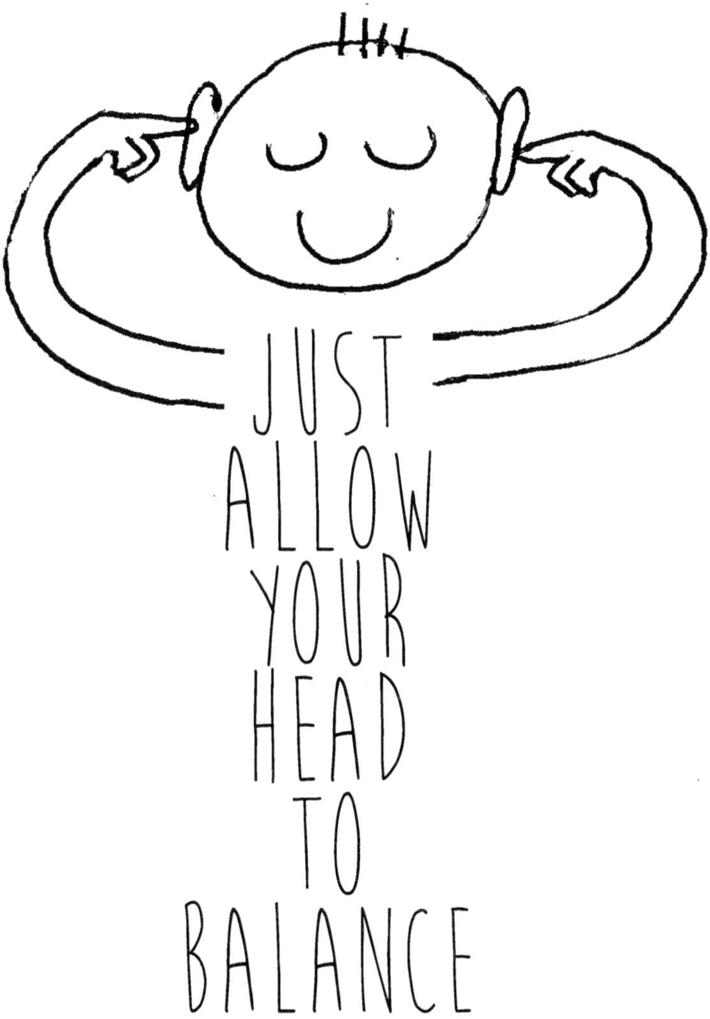

SHOULDERS

Think of your shoulder girdle as a yoke, like the ancient Asian cultures used to transport pails of water.

Allow your shoulders to gently rest on top of your rib cage.

Remember these four tips:

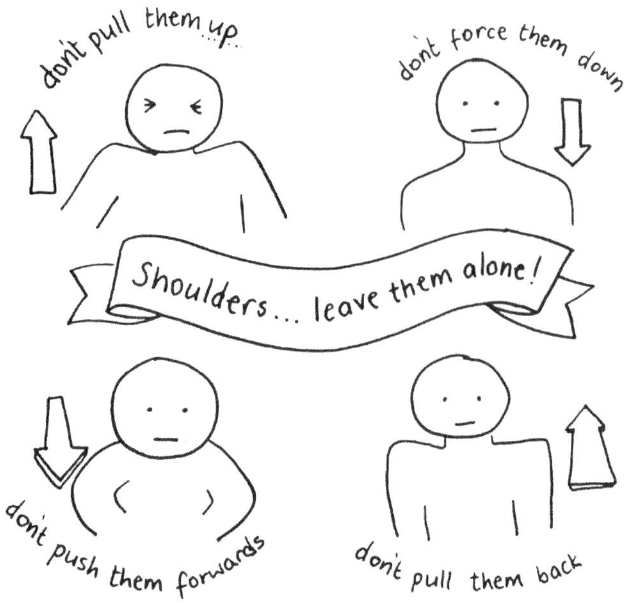

don't pull them up
don't force them down
Shoulders... leave them alone!
don't push them forwards
don't pull them back

DON'T
pull the shoulders up
force the shoulders down
push the shoulders forwards
pull the shoulders back

WHAT THEN?

LEAVE THEM ALONE!

Allow your collar bones to be long. They give important structure to the upper end of the torso. Allow your shoulder blades to float home on the back of the rib cage. Allow the humerus (long bone in the upper arm) to float into the space surrounding it within the shoulder joint.

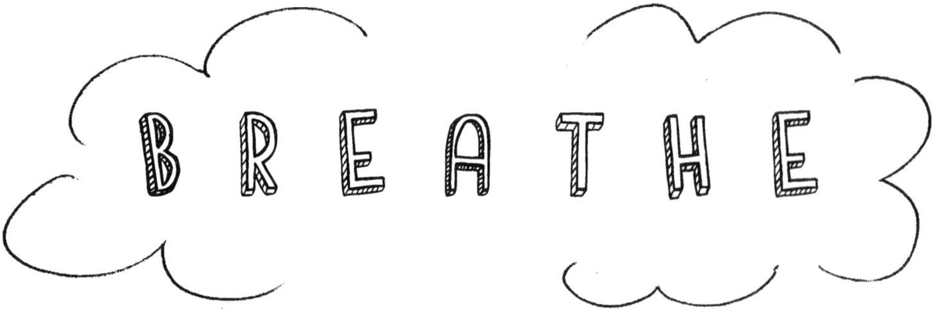

BREATHE

NOTE FROM THE AUTHOR:

Some of the directions I give are for metaphorical purposes, i.e. they help with the simple accessible overview I wish to convey. They work well in my experience with clients, so I use them here deliberately in order to help **YOU** too.

Occasionally the directions are anatomically 'poetic'. But, for now, they are the best way I know of to describe something similar to what I mean, which of course falls short of the 'hands-on' experience. As Alexander said: "Be careful of the printed matter: you may not read it as it is written down."

I ask you to bear this in mind if you notice something you disagree with, and have a suggestion not to take everything 'literally'. Creativity is the key to body compliance. As we evolve over time, our understanding of ourselves deepens and, of course, will change as our overall consciousness increases. Let's not forget, too, that we are always aiming for a more natural co-ordination. In this way we are able to improve the habitual use of ourselves with continued thought and practical application of Alexander's work.

your invitation to

CHAPTER THREE

Heads Up - How to Sit, Stand & Move with Ease

Now that we've learned what's where in our bodies, we can apply that knowledge while we 'do' something.

As an AT teacher, I often start by teaching sitting and standing, as they are simple activities that feature frequently in all of our daily lives. It's important to get these basics right to improve our functioning during our waking hours.

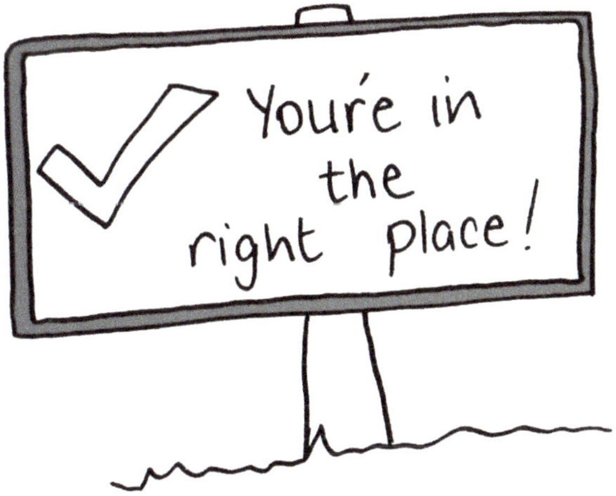

Does learning how to stand, sit and move with ease, sound good? You're in the right place.

Find somewhere quiet where you won't be disturbed. If you can be looking out of a window to an enjoyable view, that's helpful. If you can watch the birds in the garden or see other people walking by, it helps to keep your attention alive and in the present moment.

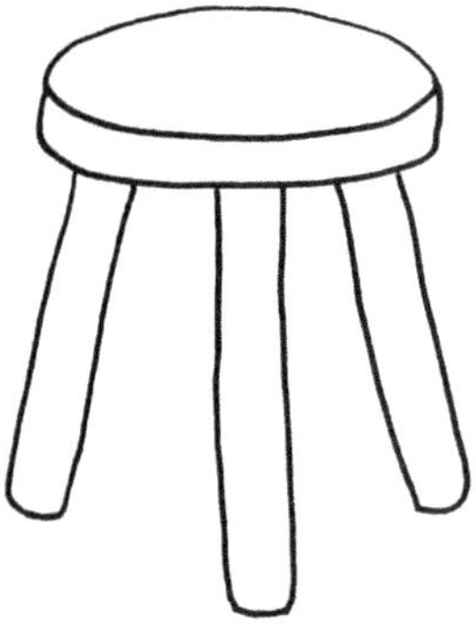

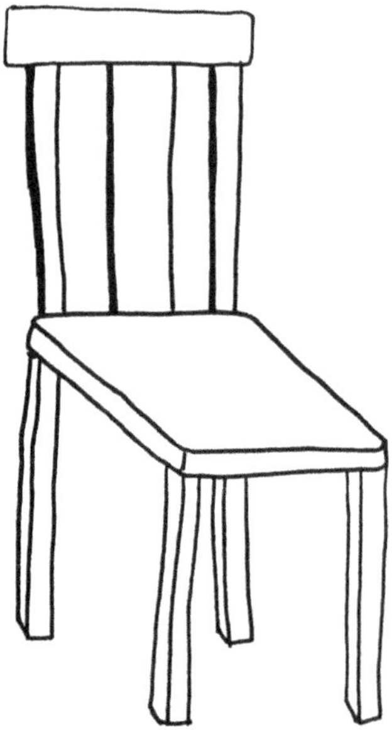

Find yourself a dining or kitchen chair or a stool. A flat, wooden seat is ideal. If this isn't possible, place a yoga block on top of a moulded seat to give you a flat surface.

Stand in front of the chair facing the window and enjoy the view. Now, without changing anything, **NOTICE** where your body weight is being distributed on your feet right now. Which foot is doing more?

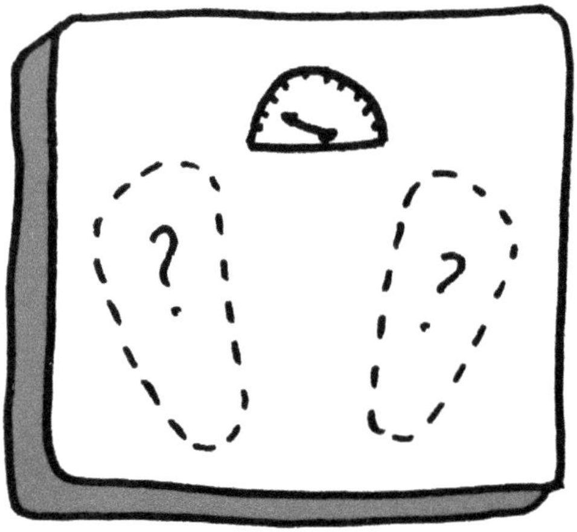

Now be **CLEAR** in your thinking about what **YOU** want to happen in **YOUR** body. Nature would prefer us to be in balance, in other words sharing our body weight evenly between both feet. This is **OPTIMAL**, and most efficient with our energy.

Request this now of your body. Just observe while your whole self reorganises itself to accommodate your wish.

You're moving towards a more **NATURAL** state and on the way to being grounded.

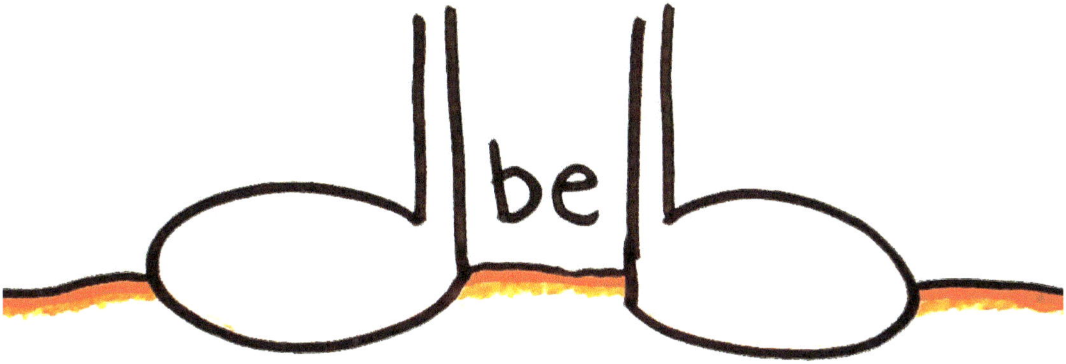

grounded

In an ideal world, each foot, as you know from the whistle-stop anatomy tour in the previous chapter, would be making FULL contact equally between these three points of contact:

The base of the big toe, the base of the little toe, and the heel.

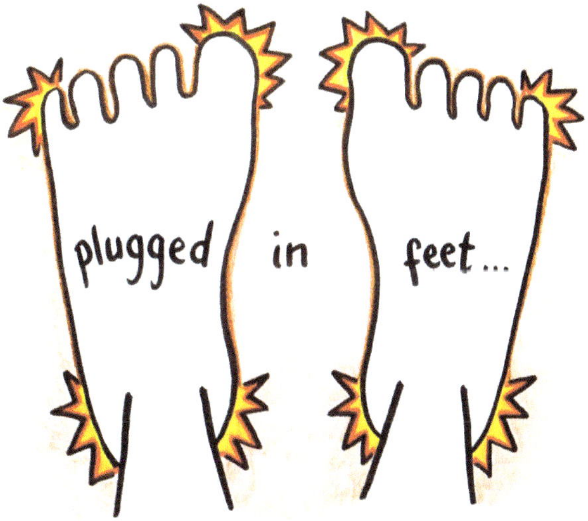

So plug them into the ground, and fully receive its support to reveal ...

happy marvellous feet

... happy to support you fully in a springy elastic fashion.

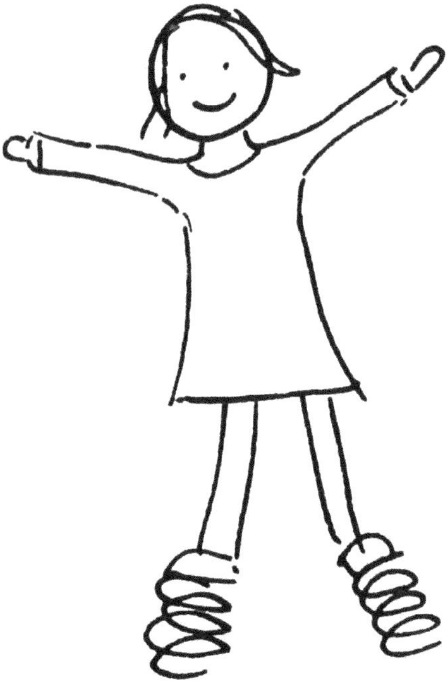

The arches of the foot are domed from front to back and also domed from side to side in nature. Make sure you're not flattening yours out.

Just let **GRAVITY** rest the foot fully on the ground and allow your postural reflexes to work. **MUCH** less effort, you see!

You might have shifted on your ankles, too, during this process. This is to be expected and is a positive sign that change is taking place!
Free up your ankle joints, remembering how far they are in front of your heels. Think up off the joint and continue thinking up your whole calf, including the outer edge of the lower leg, all the way up to the knee joint.

The knee bends from the back through to the front. Let the knee-cap fall out from the hip. Now **THINK** the knees one away from the other.

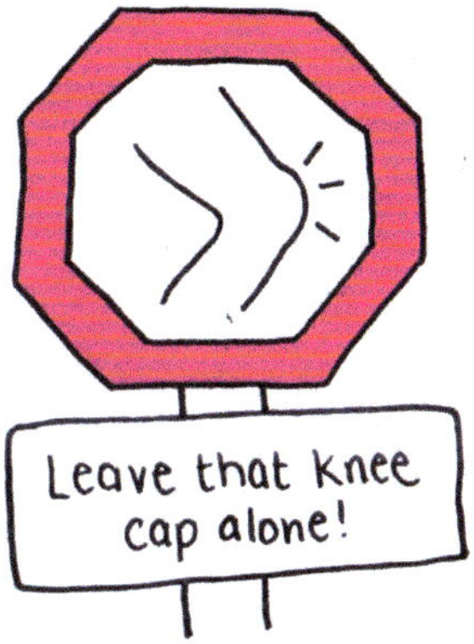

Continue thinking **UP** off the knee joint, **UP** the thigh to the hip joint.

Allow the muscles around the head of the femur (i.e. the hip joint) to release the leg from the pelvis. Remember the hip joint as being almost in the knicker line. (Yes, it is that low down, and that far away from your brain! It takes a little while for the message to reach the right place and be actioned, so have patience! It will happen; trust yourself.)

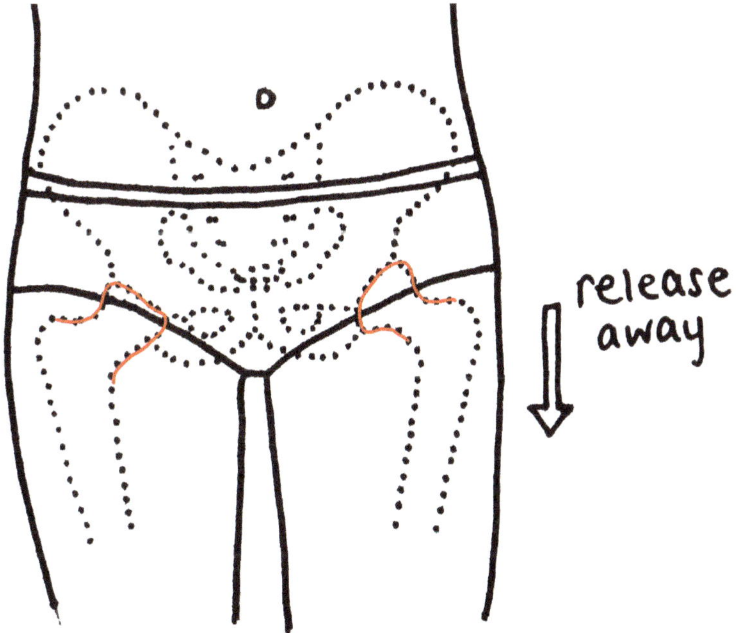

Now let your pelvis be the weight that it is and **HANG** from the head like the anchor it is to the lower end of the torso.

This bony structure is HEAVY and opposes the weight of the head. The antagonistic action gives the spine its flexibility and spring, so it's **ESSENTIAL** to allow it to be the weight, height, depth and breadth that it **ACTUALLY** is. Are you doing that?

Let your tummy out ('Let your tummy out' means it is relaxed, **NOT** pulled in, but not forced out either.)... **BREATHE** ... and now let's consider the spine.

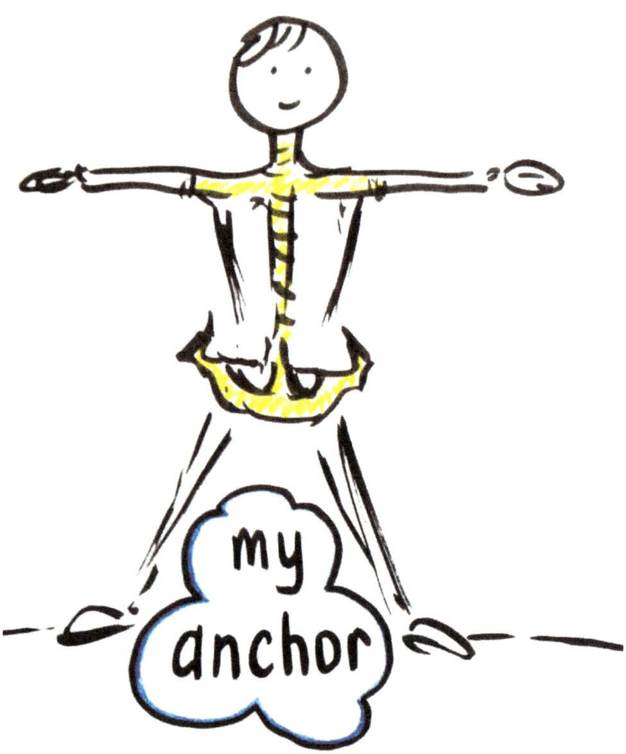

Allow the curves

Direct your tail bone to the ground below you. Get a sense of your head lengthening up your **WHOLE** spine. Allow the curves. Trust that the spine knows how it would like to organise itself and just observe while your **CLEAR INTENTIONS** are being actioned by your compliant body.

The **HEAD** is being released by the top of the spine. Do you remember where that is? That's right, all the way up between the ears, and behind the eyes. Make sure your thinking is **HIGH** enough up your spinal column.

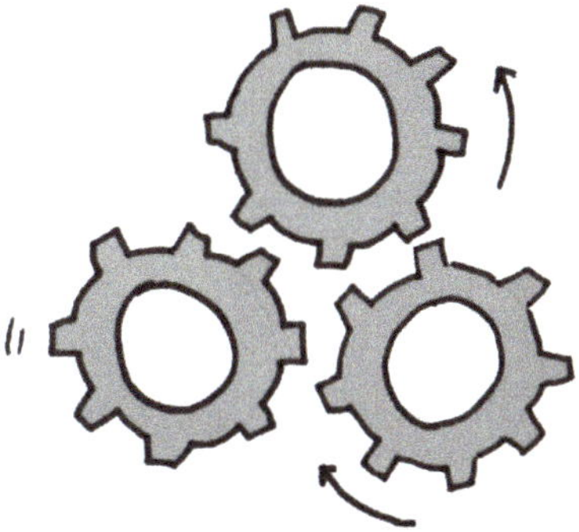

Think of the top three vertebrae as little wheels constantly turning, **ALWAYS** sending the **HEAD** away from the top of the spine. You want the top of your spine to be flowing directly UP to the ceiling.

The **HEAD** then falls **UPWARDS**, **AWAY** from the top joint (the atlanto-occipital joint) and **FORWARDS** in relation to the spine.

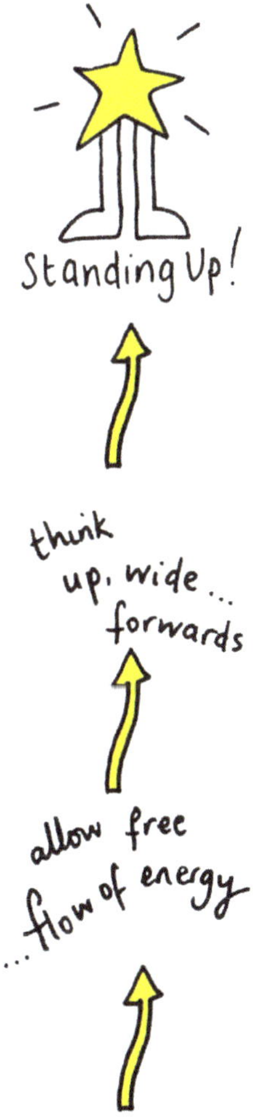
Standing Up!
think
up, wide ...
forwards
allow free
... flow of energy

breathe! ... this is really good work.

THINK shoulders one away from the other.

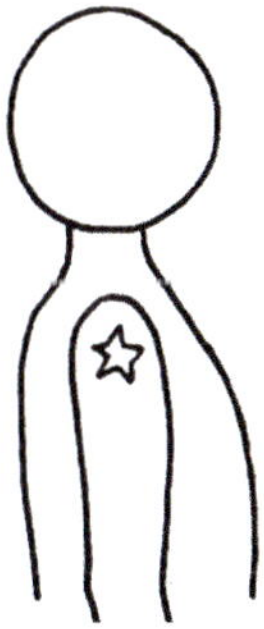
☆ shoulders hang freely
☆ check where yours are
☆ allow them to return 'home'

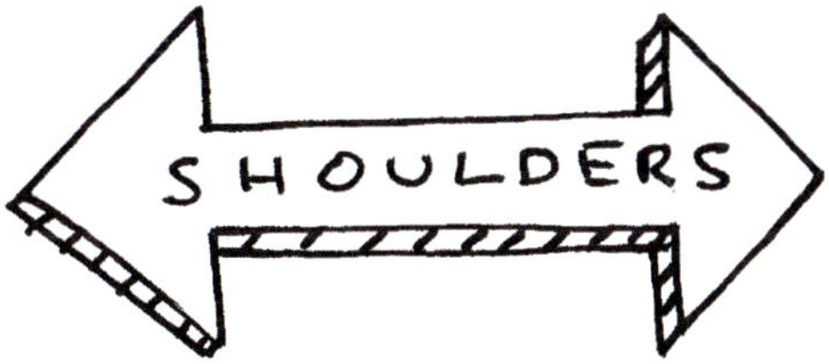
SHOULDERS

Now a little recap ... Plug in feet, think **UP** off ankles, **UP** calves, allow knees to be forwards, and away from each other, **ON THE LATCH**, soft and available for movement. Think UP off the hips. Send the head away from the top of the spine.

Now **FOLD** to sitting!

The chair feels like a **LONG WAY DOWN** when you leave your spine intact!

Many people feel very vulnerable and alarmed during this process.

It's normal!
You are moving in an unusual way.
Expect some accompanying 'different' sensations to arise.

The trouble is we have created a **WAIST** where we often interrupt the efficient spine.

Incorrectly, we articulate an unnatural joint!

KEEP YOUR SPINE LONG
to avoid waist trouble!

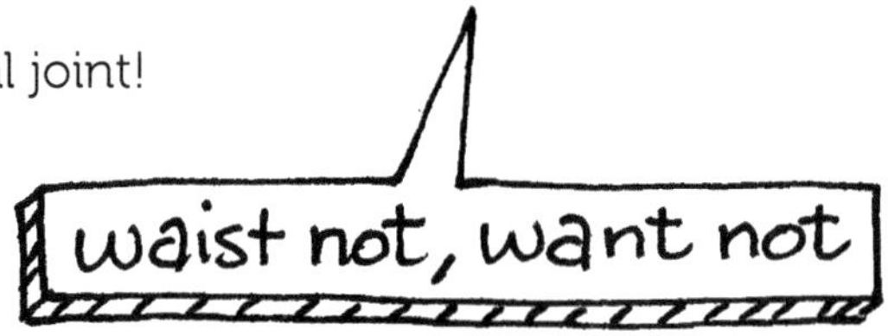

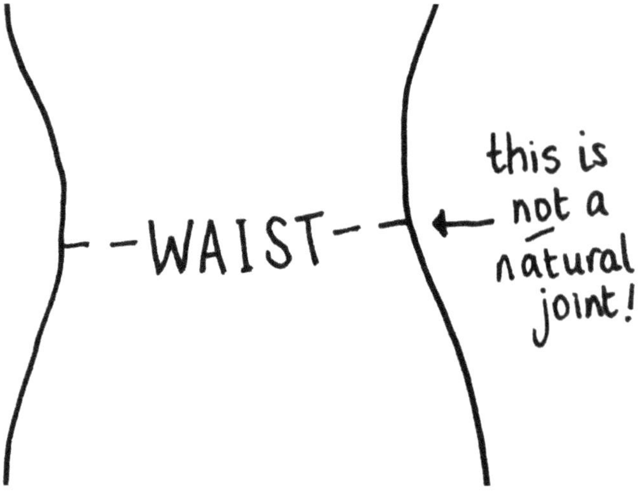

Are you sitting comfortably?

When you arrive at your seat, allow your seat bones to connect with the chair or yoga block **FULLY**.

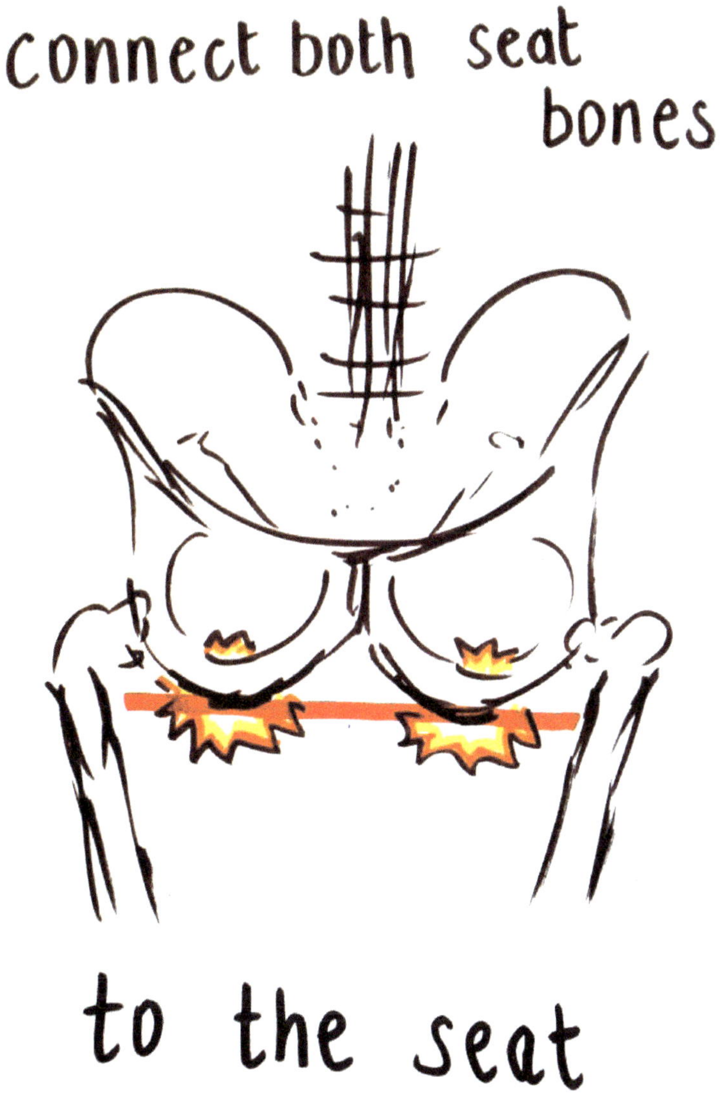

Notice if you have a favourite seat bone.

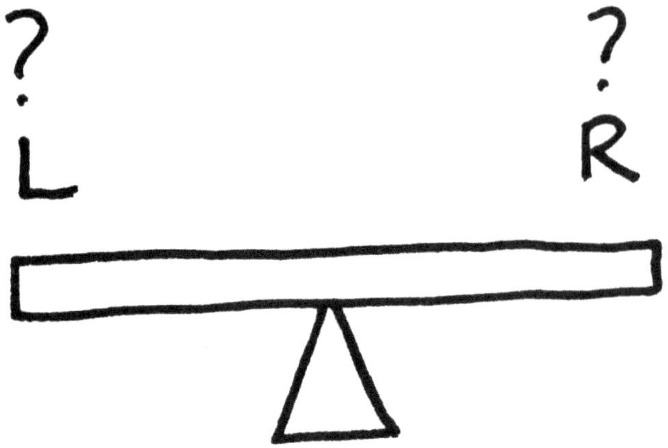

Now ask your body to reorganise itself such that BOTH seat bones are sharing the weight of your torso and head evenly. The seat bones are **ROCKER** shaped, so remember there's no fixed place, but you want a strong connection. I like to think of the seat bones as a **TWO-PIN PLUG**.

Truly accept the **FULL** support of the chair through this positive connection.

Your feet also still want to be 'plugged in', so to speak. Make sure you are continuing to allow the feet to fully contact the ground again as before, connecting:

the base of the big toe
the base of the little toe
and the heel.

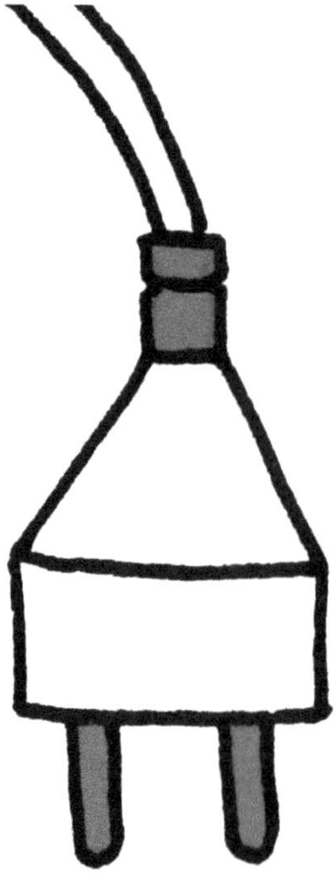

Sitting

When you are sitting, your foot wants to be directly under your knee, if possible. This allows the tibia and fibula an opportunity to lend their bony structural support to the knee joint and thigh.

Ideally, hips are higher than the knees when we're sitting, helping gravity to act on the knees, gently encouraging them out from the hips and towards the ground.

Think of releasing the leg **OUT** from the pelvis, and the leg away from the hip socket.

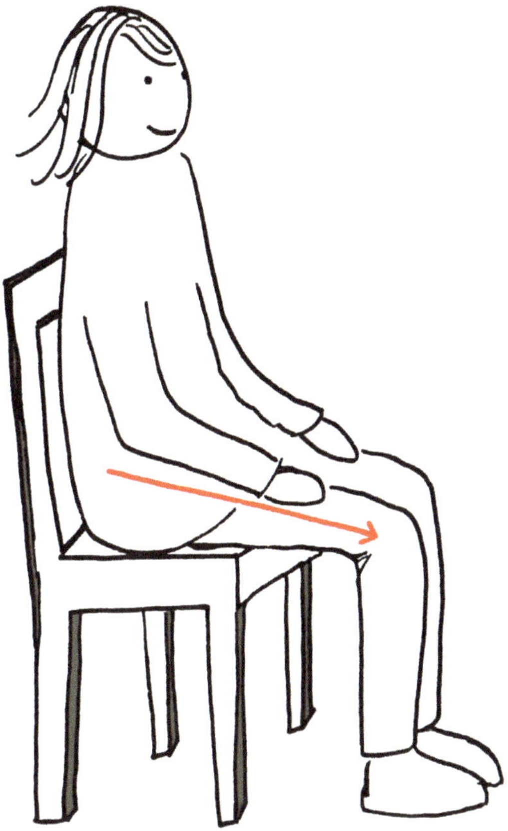

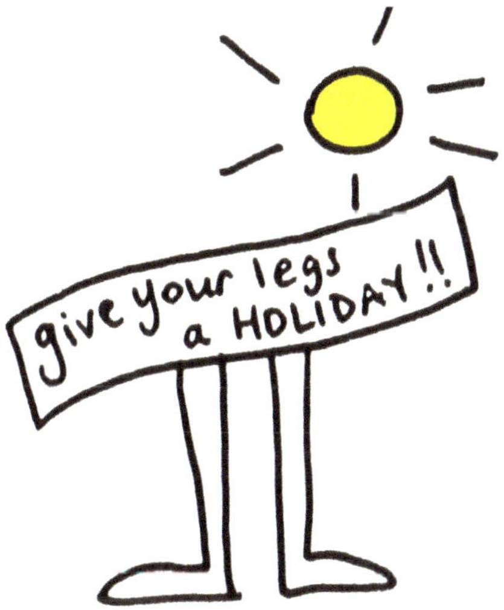

Your legs are on holiday from taking the weight of the torso right now!

When we're sitting, the torso is upright in its carriage, naturally. How is yours doing right now?

Let's investigate and see if we can improve matters!

Direct your tailbone to the ground below you. Your pelvis is anchoring you to the chair and your seat bones are evenly sharing your body weight.

Think width to the back of the pelvis. Let your tummy out ... **BREATHE**. ('Let your tummy out' means it is relaxed, **NOT** pulled in, but not forced out either.)

breathe!

Let your vertebrae organise themselves into their appropriate natural curves. It's tempting to tilt the pelvis according to our personal habit preference. This either collapses the spine encouraging the habitual '**SLUMP**' or it overarches the lumbar spine, which **LOOKS** very smart and is a common misconception of 'good posture'. Like the sergeant major, shoulders are forced back but this requires **EFFORT** and is **NOT** natural!

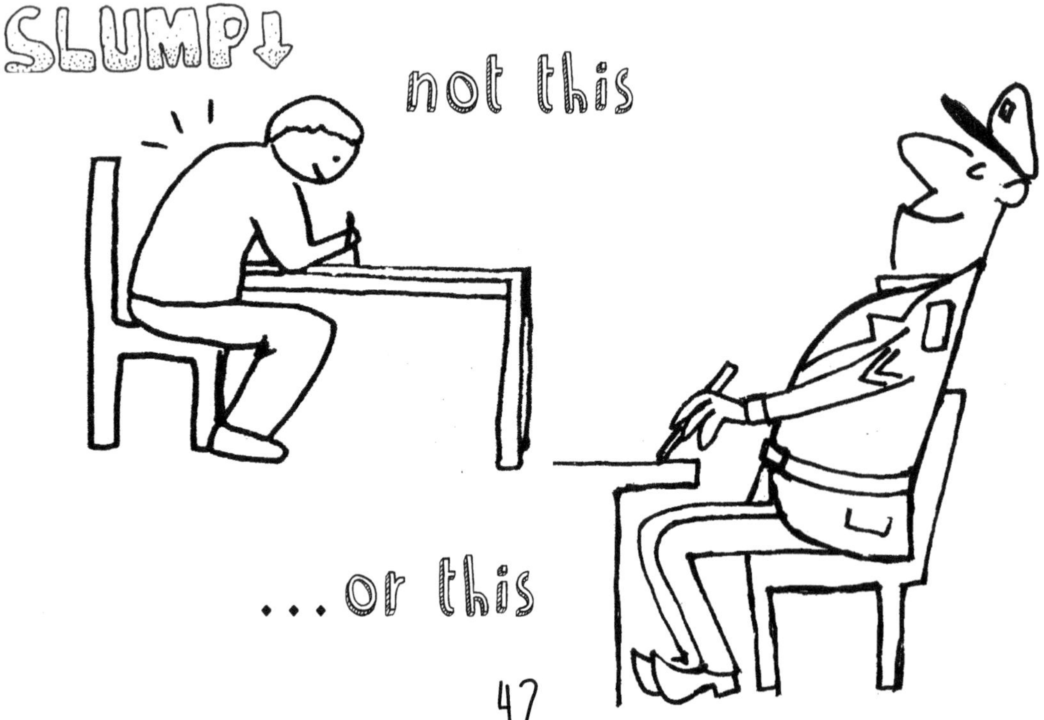

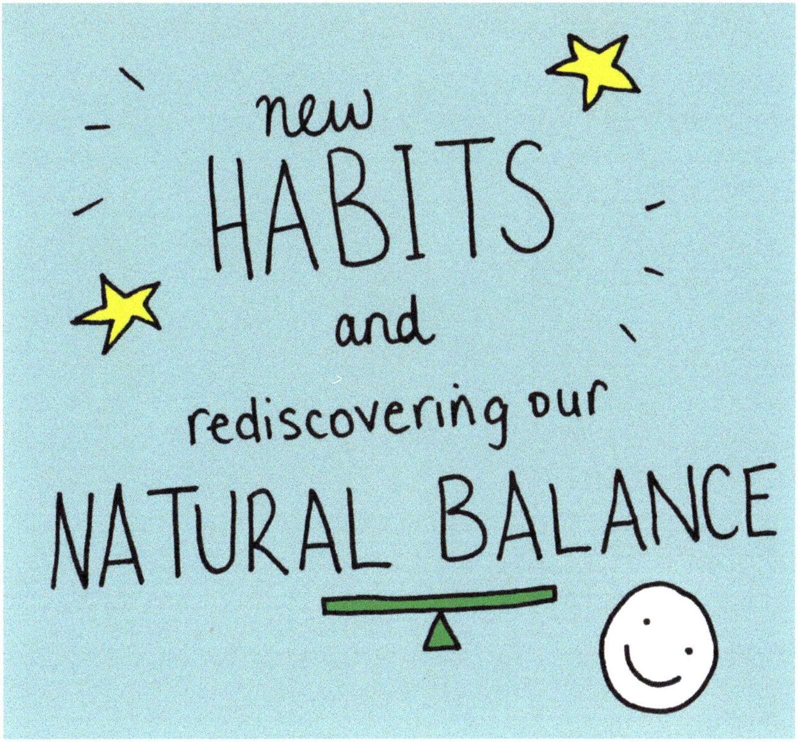

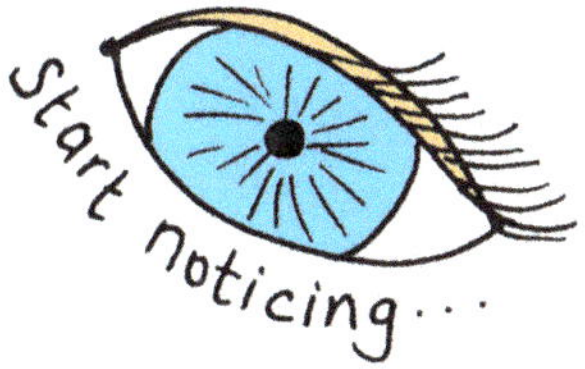

Springy elastic support is provided by a lengthening spine organised into its appropriate curves. It looks **BEAUTIFUL**, very graceful, easy, and is comfortable for long periods of time when you get used to practising 'Alexandered' thinking!

THINKING and expanding your awareness to get out of unhelpful habits is the key

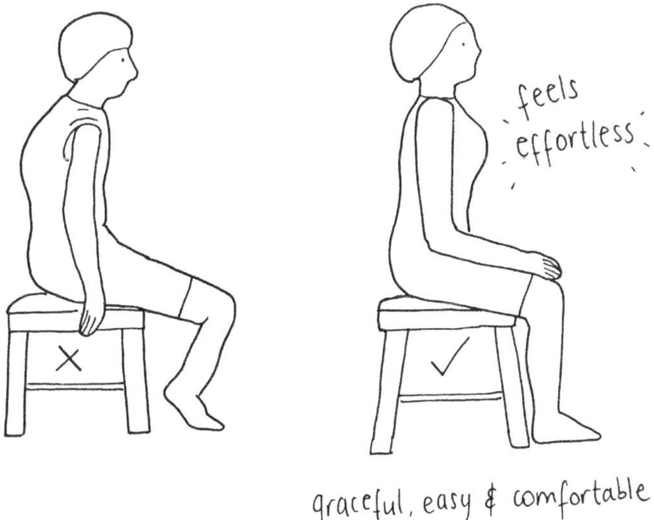

.And, of course, the more we practise this art, the better we get at doing it. Like learning any skill, practice is the key to success. **NOT** trying harder, however! Rather, **SUBTRACTING** our habits is the name of the game here, revealing our latent natural ability that was quietly waiting all along.

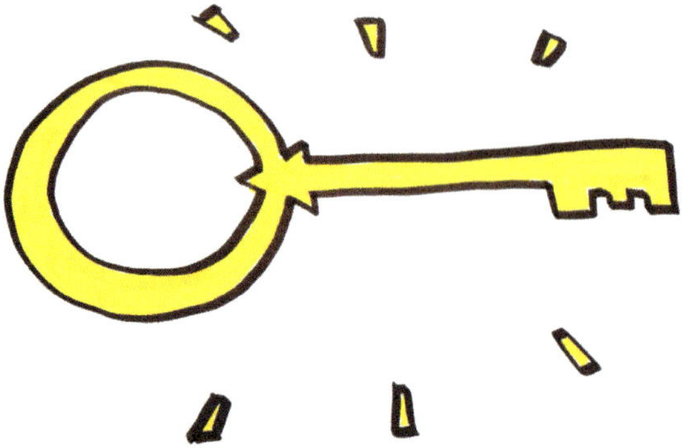

> All you'll get is the absence of what you had.
>
> **Marj Barstow**

All we have to do is get out of our own way!

Often, we get a glimpse of this accompanied by a thought that goes something like this:

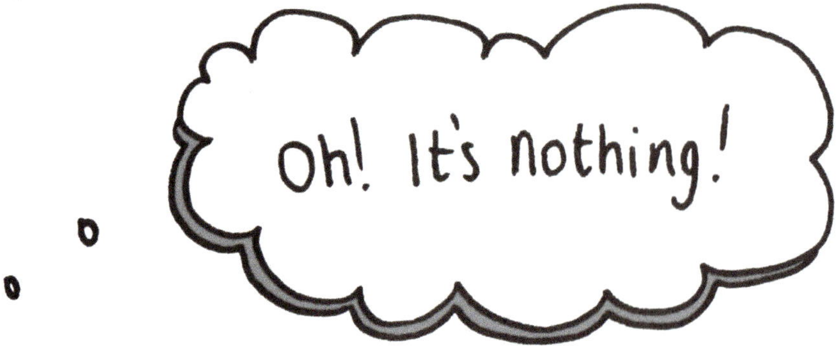

Now where were we ...?

Yes, thinking about the spine. You've made sure the tailbone is directed to the ground below; you've allowed the spinal column to organise itself back into its natural curves.

Now, get a sense of your head lengthening up your **WHOLE** spine, sending it away and **FORWARDS** from the atlanto-occipital joint (behind the eyes and between the ears).

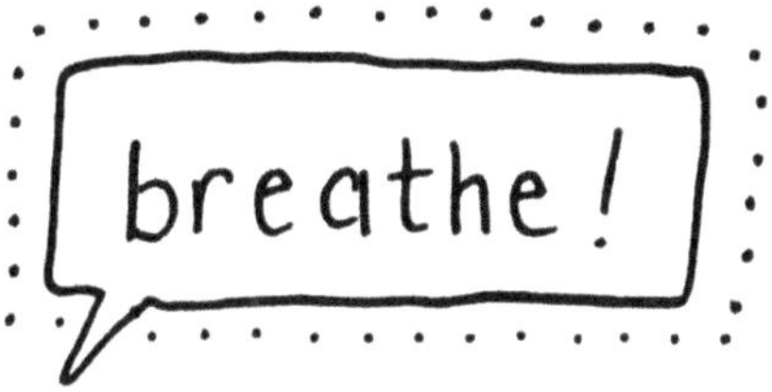

Now get your thinking cap on again. Free your ankles, knees and hips. Think UP off them all and allow your spine to release the head again.

The head leads your body **UP** and forwards. You pivot from your **FREE** hips and move freely. Keep lengthening your whole spine **UP** – continue to breathe – keeping all your natural hinges fully available to you during this movement, and allow your tummy out.

Experiment here: allow free flow of energy and let your body follow your head thinking **UP, WIDE, FORWARDS** all the time, all the way, until you find yourself standing on your own two feet again!

What happened?

Did you get stuck somewhere?

If so, try the process again from sitting. Ask yourself where the thinking stopped previously. Did doubt step in? Doubt will stop you in your tracks every time! This is usually accompanied by a thought something like this:

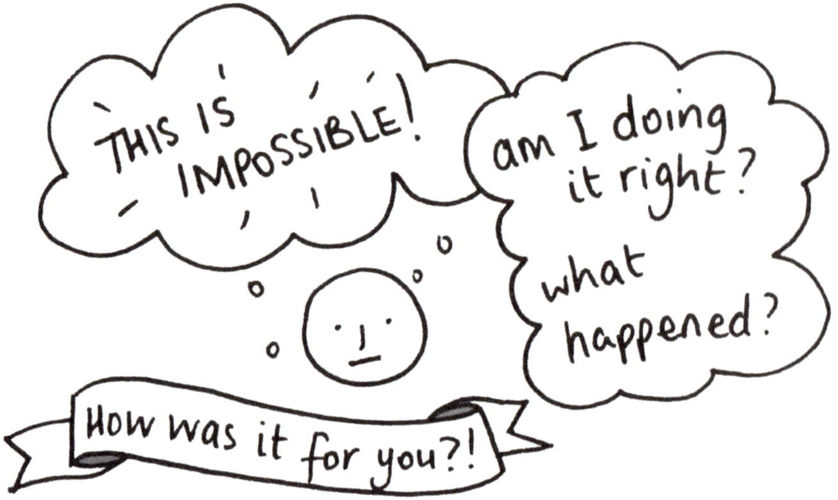
THIS IS IMPOSSIBLE!
am I doing it right?
what happened?
How was it for you?!

So I ask you:

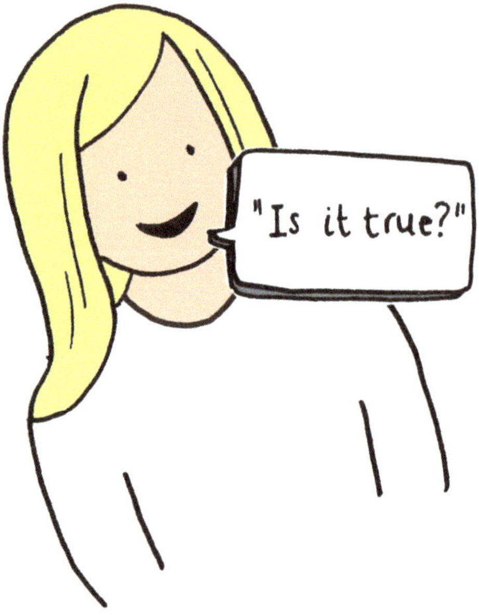
"Is it true?"

Experiment again ...

What happens THIS time?

You see – every time, our thought processes are different! And what you'll find is, IF you can suspend doubt and **ALL** your personal habits and **ONLY** apply this very simple, constructive Alexander thinking, your head will lead and your body will follow, effortlessly.

SIMPLE!

It absolutely is possible **AT SOME POINT** to attain this ability to be free of **UNDUE** tension. To have movement in all your joints all you need is:

PATIENCE & TRUST

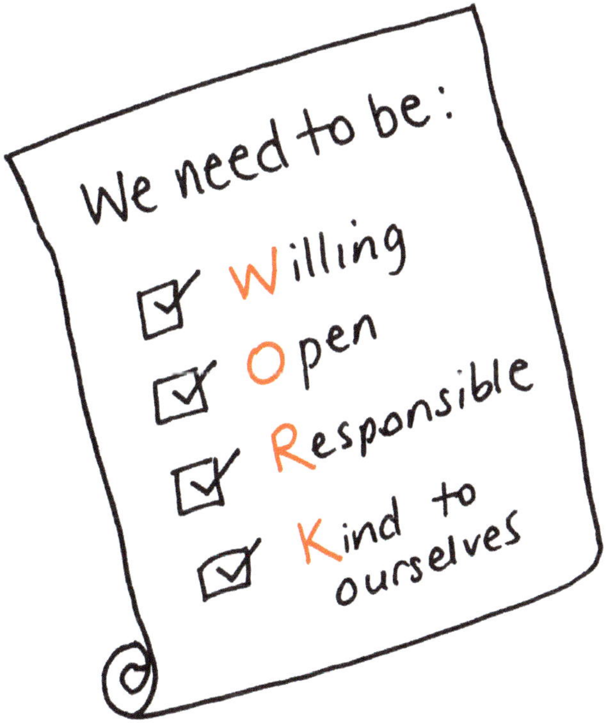
We need to be:
Willing
Open
Responsible
Kind to ourselves

It will happen. If at first you don't succeed, try again. Experiment, experiment, experiment ... discover ... learn, and this (mostly) pleasurable (but **OK**, I admit, sometimes irritating) journey builds up a **VERY** interesting and **HUGE** database of knowledge and information **ABOUT YOU**!

We can begin to start noticing all sorts of unhelpful personal habits we're often drawn into.

So don't be afraid of being wrong, there's no such thing, there is only learning, and how rich this learning is if we're prepared to be open, honest, truthful and kind to ourselves.

> Thank you so much for working such wonders on my posture. A couple of days after our last session another bit of the jigsaw fell into place and I'm just so delighted with my progress. I am completely twinge free and am constantly using all the little manoeuvres you taught me. The way I stand, sit, walk, lie and turn has changed forever!
>
> **Dr Nicola Kirk – Lead Consultant Microbiologist at Ashford and St Peter's Hospital**
> **Presented with 20 years of back pain**

CHAPTER FOUR

THE ALEXANDER TECHNIQUE SEMI-SUPINE – HOW TO BE A THOUGHTFUL LAYABOUT!

After all that hard mental 'work' in the previous chapter, now comes your reward! The gift of Alexander Technique semi-supine. In simple terms it means a nice lie down!

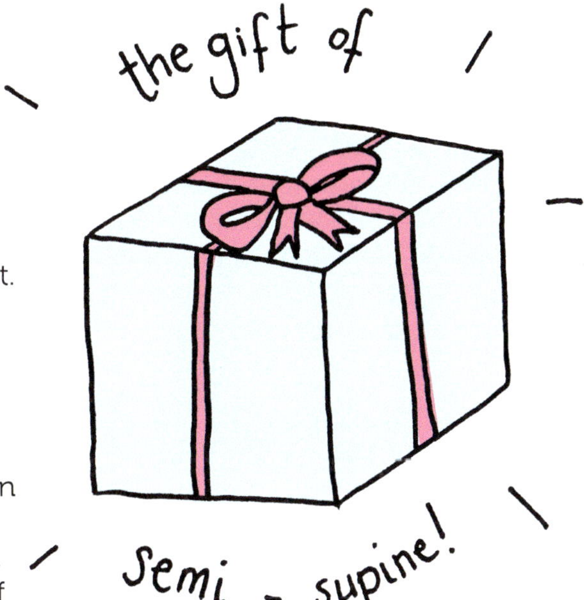

It is not 'doing nothing', however! This is a mindful, nurturing practice that gives many benefits to you **IF** you can allow yourself the time to actually do it.

We often resist this step, coming up with all sorts of 'valid' excuses, such as "I don't have time", "I've got far too much to do" and so on – the sort of self-sabotage we justify to ourselves on a daily basis. It does become easier to allow this step into our lives over time, once we realise the cost to ourselves if we **DON'T** make the time available. I would even go so far as to say that it's one of the most important and beneficial aspects of the Alexander Technique, especially at the beginning of the learning process.

In just **20 minutes** you can be fully restored, energised and able to continue your day much more effectively as a result.

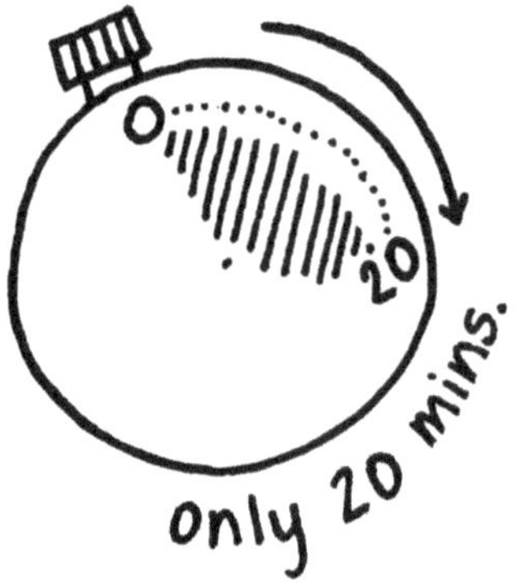

Give yourself a pat on the back, too, for allowing this special 'me' time. It's totally responsible and very much a part of this practice of 'looking after yourself'.

Living a hectic modern life usually entails an excessively demanding schedule much of the time. Humans are not meant to endure these conditions for such long periods of time, day in, day out, year in, year out. So, before we burn out, let's add back in some 'down time', which brings some balance back into our bodies and minds.

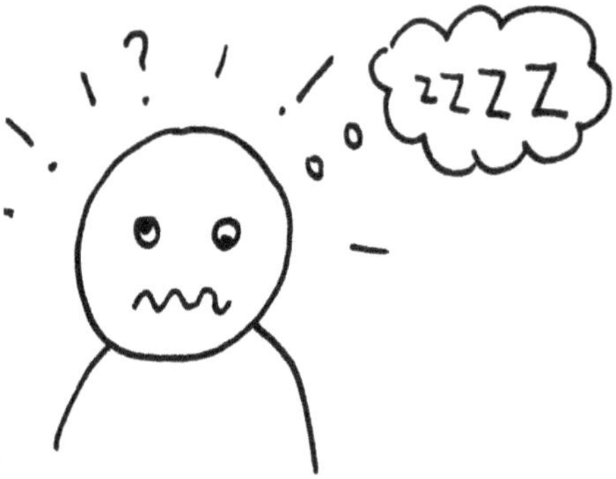

Sometimes my clients immediately fall asleep when we get to the semi-supine part of the lesson. It's quite common! It just shows how chronically tired we are. Sleep deprived and mentally overloaded, our senses are overstimulated, and our natural resources are overextended and propped up, often by artificial means, such as caffeine, alcohol or prescription drugs.

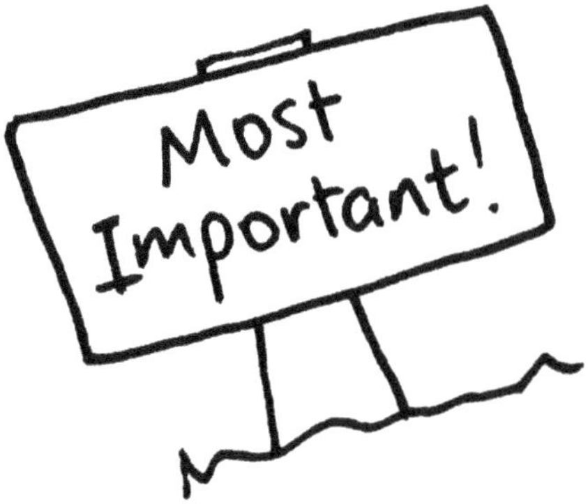

So when we **STOP** we fall asleep or sometimes we only stop when we become physically ill. The body forces us to take a breather that way.

To be in good health, we need balance, we need to be physically active and get enough exercise, we need adequate sleep every night, and we need a healthy balanced diet. Now I'm delighted to add to your repertoire THIS practice of constructive rest.

Why is it good for me?

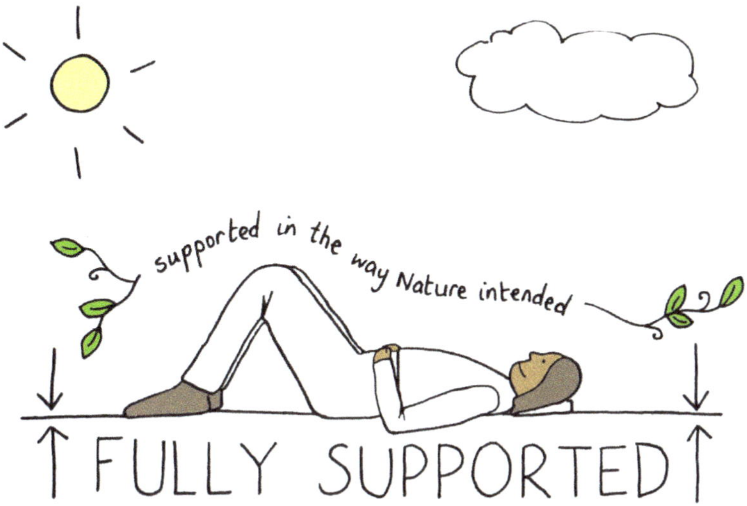
supported in the way Nature intended
FULLY SUPPORTED

When lying down in the Alexander Technique semi-supine, the body is **FULLY** supported by the floor. The body is in a completely different relationship with gravity than if you were sitting or standing. The weight of the head is alleviated from the spinal column. Its weight is fully taken by the paperback books it is resting on. The spine gets an opportunity to decompress. The vertebral discs can take this opportunity to reabsorb fluid from the surrounding tissues, improving their shock-absorbing properties once again.

As the brain is aware that the body is well supported, the muscles are more able to lengthen and release unnecessary tension as it is deemed 'safe' to do so.

It is very calming for your whole organism to be allowed to benefit from this supported state. You are lying in a position of 'mechanical advantage'. Your skeletal frame is supporting you in the way that nature intended.

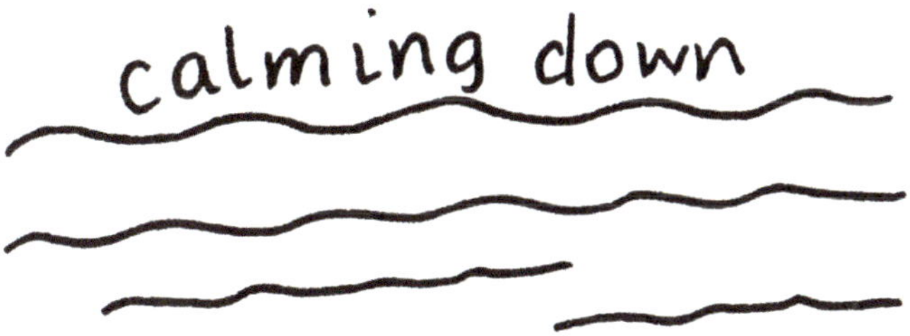
calming down

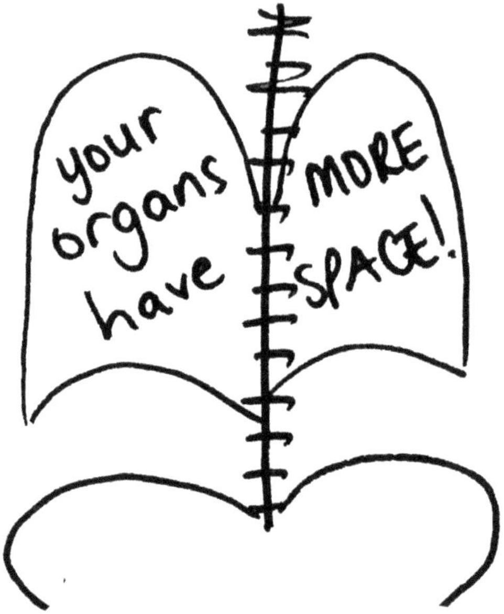

Mental noise quietens down. The business of just 'being' can begin. All our systems welcome the break from the constant cycle of 'busy-ness' that normally accompanies our waking hours.

Digestion can recommence; the circulatory system benefits from the supported state and moves more freely as tension is released; and internal space is increased as you expand into something approaching your full natural size and dimensions. Similarly, the lymphatic system can become active; breathing calms and deepens, allowing more oxygen into the system. The nervous system calms down.

The abdominal organs are able to function more efficiently too, enjoying their increased internal space to go about their duties.

So, the benefits are huge, and this restorative rest is well worth the 20 minutes set aside to indulge in it. The body begins to heal itself as it has a chance to do so.

AND IT'S FREE!

Sometimes we forget that the best things in life are free!

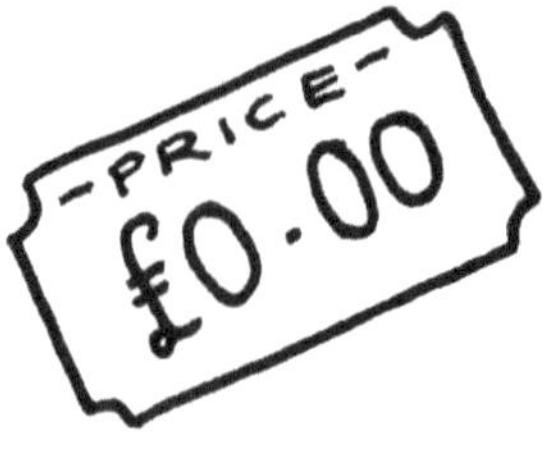

Incidentally, if you don't have 20 minutes, use the time that you do have – even one or two minutes can still be helpful.

How do we practise constructive rest?

Find a quiet room or place where you won't be disturbed for the duration of this time. Wear loose clothing that you don't mind lying down in. Switch off your mobile phone/telephone and take this time. It's important to make sure you are warm and comfortable.

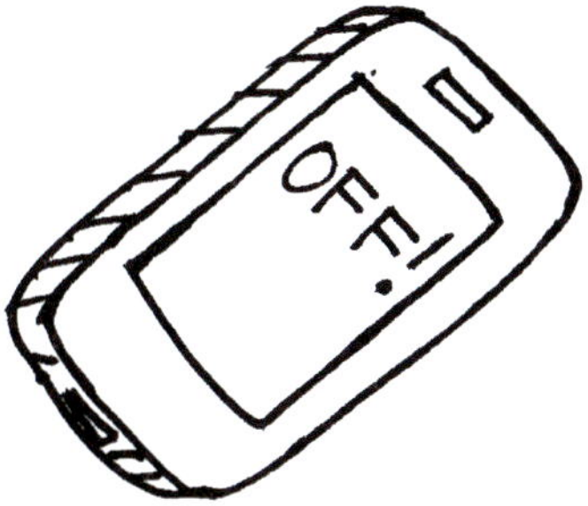

Lie on a rug or a carpeted floor. If you don't have carpet, lie on a yoga mat. You'll need a few paperback books to place under your head, or a yoga block.

Let's approach this practice consciously, so we'll learn the art of getting into and out of semi-supine safely.

Stand in balance, as discussed in Chapter 3. **BREATHE!** Now come down onto one knee. Take your time, all the while breathing, and explore this movement with curiosity.

When you feel ready, bring your other knee down. Now, slowly bring your torso forwards so you're coming onto all fours. Rock back towards your heels, then drop down onto your elbows. Turn your eyes to the right and let your head follow. Your body now wants to follow your head. Turn onto your right side and roll onto your back.

As I write, it's a gorgeous sunny day in June. I'm lying on the grass and looking up. I have a view of a cobalt blue sky; my pear tree contrasting shiny bright green leaves with gnarled, moss-covered branches arching over me. There are one or two fluffy white clouds in the sky. Birds are tweeting, butterflies fluttering around...Bliss!
If you're experiencing a similar day – go outside to do your semi-supine; even better to be in nature if possible.

Your head is supported by the paperback books or yoga block. As a general rule, too many books is better than too few. You want your neck to be comfortable. You don't want your head to tip back.

Your knees are aiming at the sky; your hands resting gently on your abdomen.

Now, you're just going to observe yourself in this position and allow your whole body to begin to unwind. Ask your body to release into length from the crown of your head to the tips of your toes.

You are allowing your whole body to make contact with the ground. Gravity is working on the whole of you, pulling you in that direction. There's nothing to 'do', there's nothing to 'think' ... you're just being here now, fully with yourself in this present moment.

Invite your neck to free itself from any unnecessary tension. Allow your head to flow away from the top of your spine. Your head is lengthening away from your tailbone, which is flowing in the opposite direction.

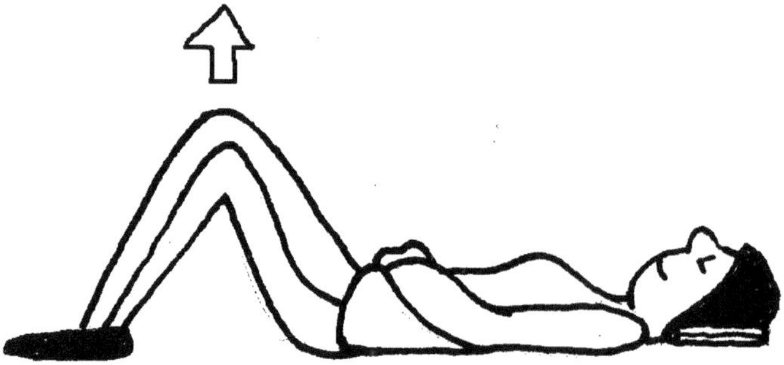

Breathe, blink gently and notice where your body is making contact with the ground.

The back of your head, the backs of your shoulders, parts of your spine – which parts? The back of your pelvis – how is it contacting the floor? The three points of contact on each foot. Each elbow. Breathe.

Invite your shoulders to flow one away from the other. Allow your collar bones to be long across the width of your upper torso. Let the shoulder blades gently float 'home' onto the back of the rib cage.

Remember, these are just mental directions and requests, **NOT** muscular actions. You remain a silent witness to the changes occurring in your body, letting them all 'be'.

If any strange sensations come up, explore them with curiosity. What are they

saying to you?
Invite your neck to free itself again. Continue sending your head away from the top of your spine. Keep on sending your tailbone away from your head in the opposite direction.

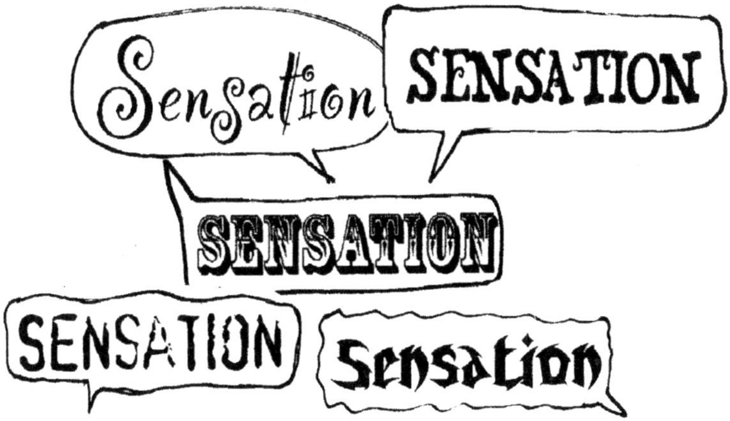

Accept gravity's friendly, gentle pull towards the ground with your **WHOLE BODY.** Breathe.

Your knees are still flowing up to the ceiling, away from each other and out from beautifully free hips.

Ask your right shoulder to make a lengthening diagonal connection to your left hip ... across the front of your body **AND** the back of your body. Now ask your left shoulder to discover a lengthening diagonal connection with the right hip, across the front **AND** the back of the body.

Notice the rise and fall of the breath.

Let your eyes float back into their sockets. Let your jaw release away from the skull. Teeth should be gently contacting each other, **NOT** clenched. Your tongue should be softly resting in the lower palate. Your soft palate is just that – **SOFT!**

Now free the neck again; let the head flow away from the top of the spine. Your entire spinal column will be pleased to be able to lengthen, widen and deepen. Knees should be floating **UP** to the ceiling.

Notice the ribs. Are they freely moving with respiration? Gently but firmly, insist on them being free to move with the breath action.

Continue this cycle of gentle attention, lightly bringing into your mind different parts of your body.

Ask your ankles to free up, knees to float up to the ceiling. Your hips are releasing from the pelvis, which is beautifully supported by the ground.
As the time for active rest comes to a close, don't speed up your thinking and rush out of it! Realise you're still lying on the ground; allow the floor to continue supporting you. Continue to ask for freedom in your neck muscles, so that your head can maintain its direction away from the top of your spine, thus allowing the spine to continue lengthening, your whole back to continue widening and knees to still flow out of free hips up towards the ceiling.

Now send your left eye around to the right side. Imagine it being curious to see the texture and colour of the surface you are lying on. **WAIT** for your neck to become free before allowing your head to follow the eyes' lead.

When the body wants to come with the head, allow it to follow. Your whole body should follow the eyes around to look almost behind you.
Naturally, you should end up on all fours again. Breathe, take your time. Now sit back on your heels. Allow your torso to return to upright. Allow your balance to come back.

Congratulations!

Breathe, then slowly bring one knee up. Wait until you feel steady! Now, when you're ready, bring the other knee up to return to standing.

You should now be replenished, restored and more springy and revitalised than you were 20 minutes ago!

> I do semi-supine every morning and it definitely has made a wonderful difference, and I really can't get through a day at the computer if I don't.
>
> **Gill Weir – Financial Controller**
> Presented with back pain, stiff neck and shoulders

Sleeping

I am often asked by my clients what the best sleeping position is.

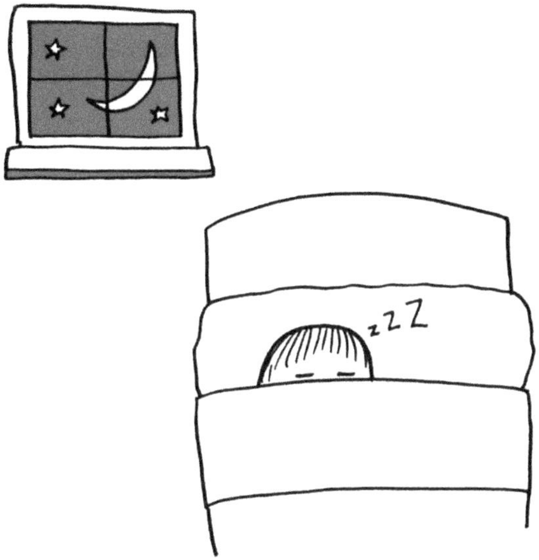

Ideally, you should sleep on your side. Make sure your pillows fill the whole width of your shoulder.

Support your head fully so that it remains in line with the rest of your spine. It can help to have a pillow between your knees and ankles, too, so your hips are supported.

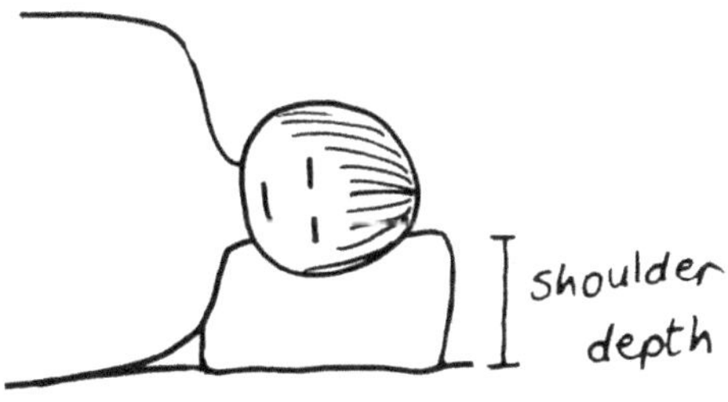

Your whole self can benefit from your attention so you are fully supported and comfortable before you doze off. This means you are conscious of **HOW** you are going to fall asleep. If we don't pay attention, we stay in tension. If you've ever woken up with a stiff neck, dead arm or similar, that's unconscious resting, which is not always restorative! So it's worth thinking about your self before you go to sleep. It will minimise the risk of a stiff neck/sore shoulders/ back pain the next day.

If you have to sleep on your back, make sure your pillow isn't too high. This encourages the neck too far forwards and out of alignment – a recipe for disaster at some point.

If you sleep on your front, ask your neck to free itself and support your head and neck. Ensure your hips, knees and ankles are free of tension. Your back wants to be able to lengthen and widen freely, too.

Any sleeping position is fine if you leave your whole body alone and free of tension. The question is: Can you? The thoughts of the day often come with us in the form of muscular tension disrupting restful sleep.

Thinking is the key **BEFORE** you go to sleep.

Good night!

What if I can't do semi-supine on the floor?

This is a valid question that is sometimes raised.

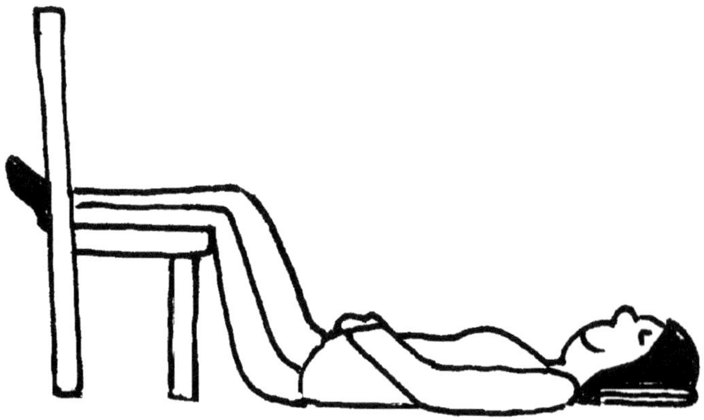

It may not be possible for some people to do semi-supine on the floor. If it's too much for health reasons to get down that low, by all means use your bed. Just **DON'T** use your pillow to support your head in semi-supine. It's too soft and won't give your brain the feedback that paperback books give.

The brain likes to know where your body is in space and it prefers positive contact to soft contact, which is less supportive. You'll still achieve some beneficial muscular release by following this advice and using your bed as the support when lying semi-supine.

Alternatively, if you can get down onto the floor, but find it hard to support your legs, support them instead on a couch or stool. This will help release hip tension while allowing your back to receive the positive support of the ground.

Pregnancy

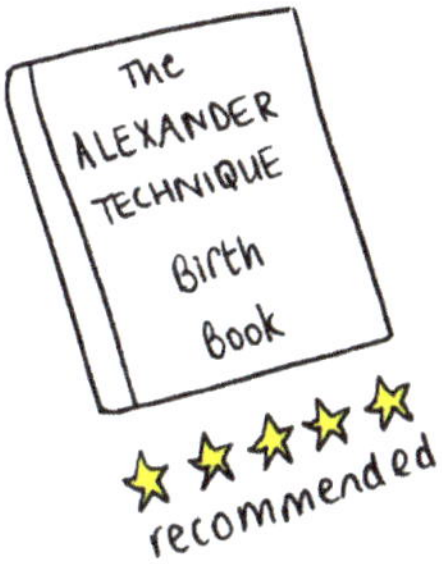

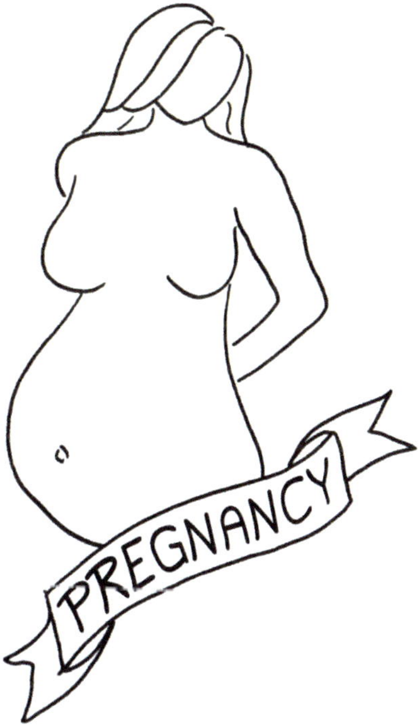

The Alexander Technique can be **SO** beneficial to mothers-to-be and their unborn babies. I highly recommend The Alexander Technique Birth Book by Ilana Machover and Angela and Jonathan Drake. It is a comprehensive guide to preparing your body for pregnancy and looking after yourself during your whole pregnancy, and includes tips on managing labour and the birth itself.

Following the birth, AT can be an invaluable support to you with the new demands of parenthood, from breast-feeding to bathing your baby. It is caring for you while you are caring for your baby. It also supports your child's development in a positive way from the beginning.

I had the pleasure of training with Ilana Machover when I attended her Eutokia course in August 2010. 'Eutokia' means happy childbirth. Alexander principles allow **YOU** to set up the optimal conditions for a natural childbirth. You achieve an overall improvement in your own balance and movement is freer. You learn how to release pressure and tension, and how to manage your body while it's undergoing many changes across the stages of pregnancy.

Semi-supine in pregnancy

At some point, probably in the second trimester, it will no longer be comfortable or advisable to lie on your back for the practice of Alexander Technique semi-supine.

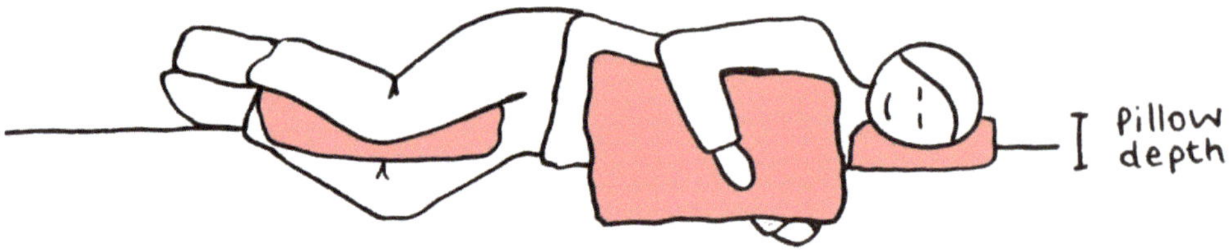

Not to worry! You can still practise active rest by lying on your side. It's a most welcome rest for your spine, as the weight of your head is taken by pillows or cushions. Fully support your head and the full width of your shoulder. You'll need a cushion between your knees and ankles to free up hips and relieve tension from them. Depending on what stage you're at, you may need a cushion under your bump, too, to support the baby's weight in this position. You'll also need to support the uppermost arm, by resting it either along your body or on another cushion or two in front of you.

The idea is to take this much needed time out to rest. It gently allows your whole body to expand, increasing the internal space. Your unborn baby **LOVES** this opportunity to stretch out a bit, not to mention your own abdominal organs.

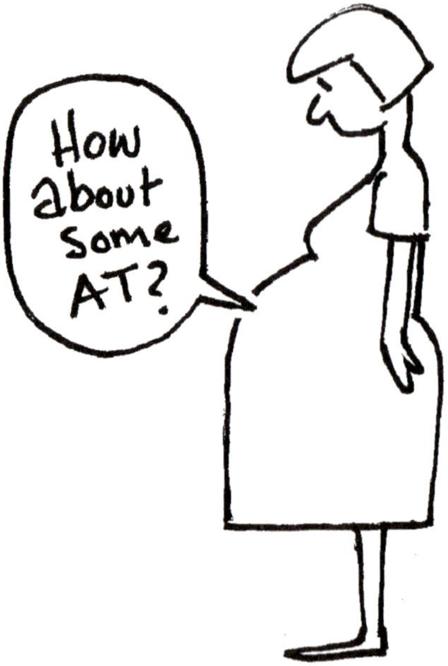

ENJOY!

CHAPTER FIVE

WORKPLACE WELLNESS

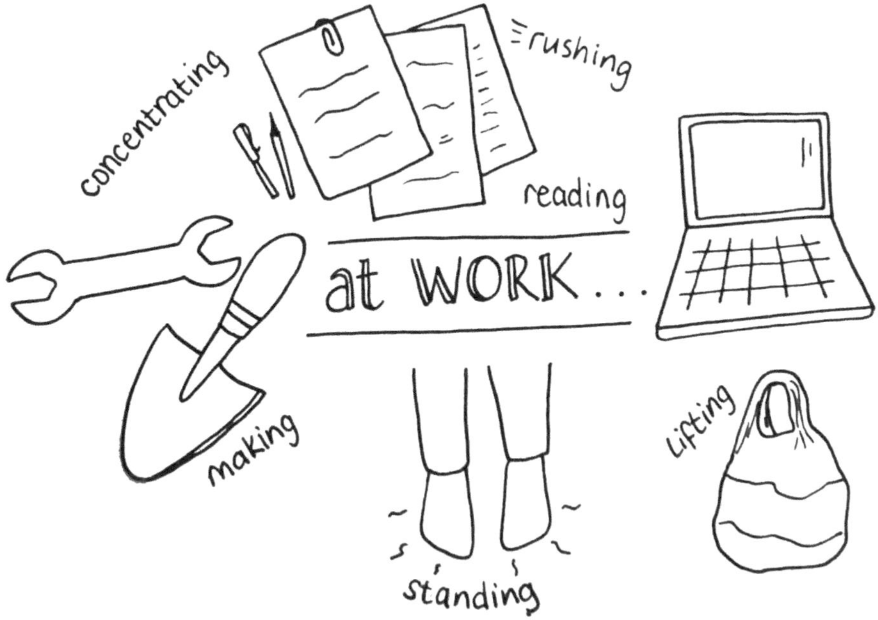

Many people pay no attention to themselves during their working hours. Indeed I was one of them! I was so conscientious that I deemed myself less important than the patients I was there to serve, the staff that I was working alongside and my employer too.

How wrong I was! And I had not even the vaguest idea that I was choosing this thinking.

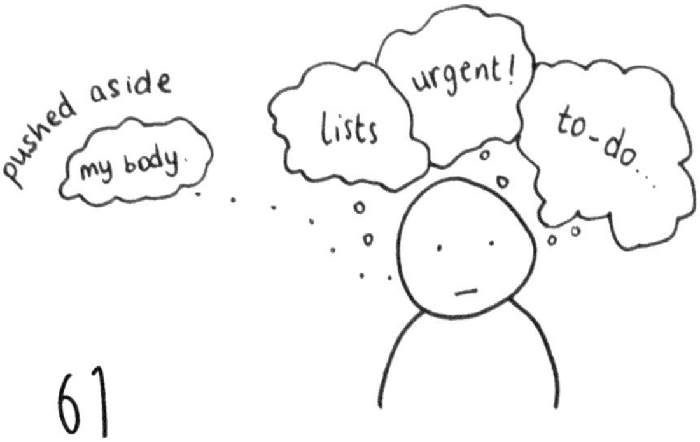

My defining moment of clarity on this issue was having a repetitive strain injury.

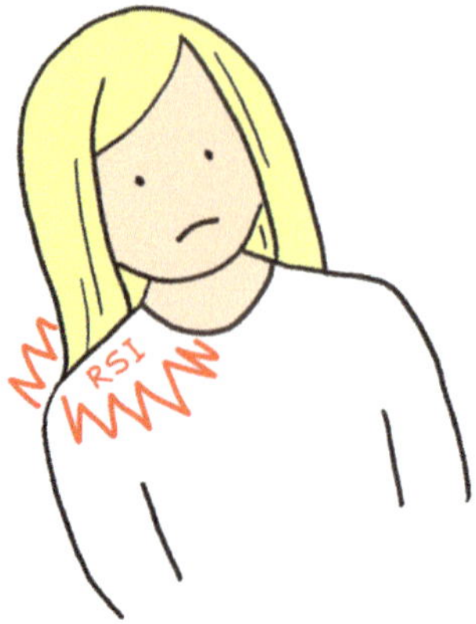
RSI

Until that moment **NOTHING** had made sense to me. I felt disconnected and disgruntled that I had a debilitating injury that just wouldn't 'go away'.
I was so unhappy about giving up my medical career, but I felt backed into a corner. It seemed the **ONLY** option available to me in order to limit any further physical injury.
Little did I know that this would lead to something **MUCH** better.
My journey taught me that I had caused the repetitive strain injury myself, albeit unwittingly.
My doctors didn't think I would heal. The advice given to me was to rest as much as possible to maintain the status quo. In other words: at best it won't get any worse!

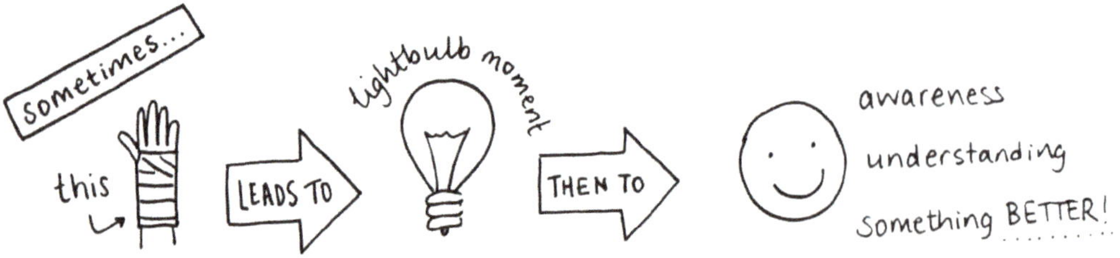
sometimes...
this
LEADS TO
lightbulb moment
THEN TO
awareness
understanding
something BETTER!

However...look at me now! I am in better shape than when I was a teenager. So what did I do? I studied the Alexander Technique and applied it to myself. Very soon my 'problem' shoulders were a thing of the past.

My issues began long before I was physically aware of them. Often problems begin at an emotional level and are reflected in the body. The body accommodates habits and patterns of misuse for long periods of time. We are blissfully unaware of the strain and tension we are putting on ourselves to cope or get through difficult circumstances. The habits to us 'feel' right and normal. The first we know is when the body is unable to accommodate unnatural behaviour any longer, and the beginnings of discomfort arrive, leading to pain and, eventually, an inability to 'function' unless we change our ways.

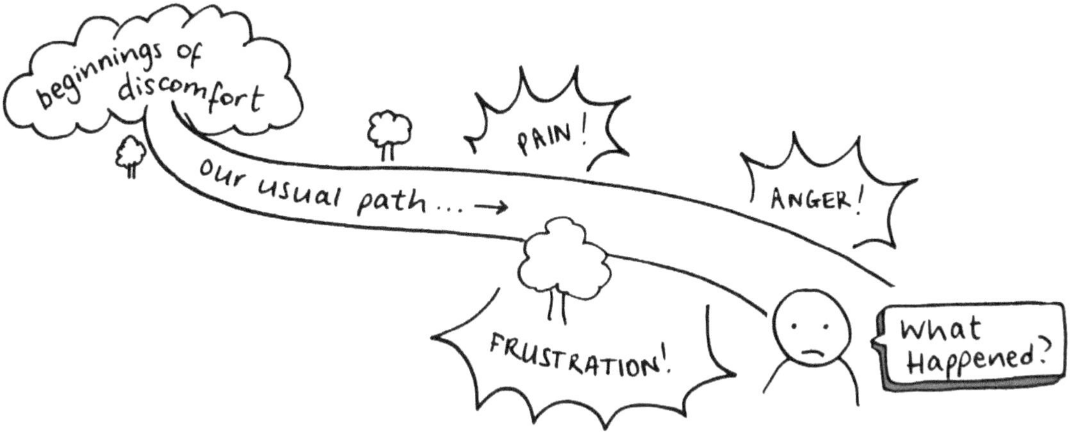

The Alexander Technique helps us to work with the body. It restores it to its natural state and allows it to heal. Our body leads the way home to a more balanced physical and emotional state.

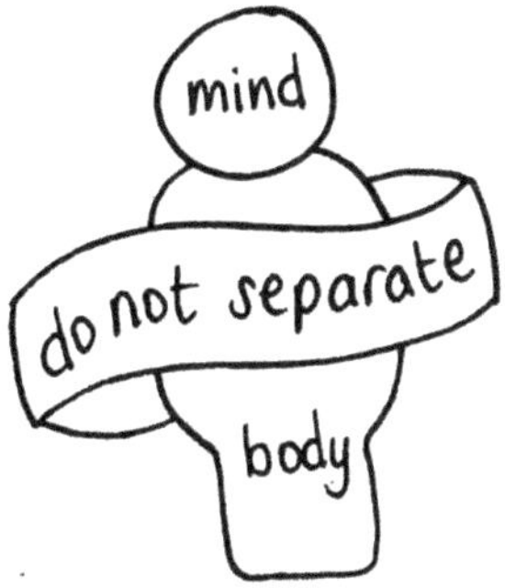

We are a psycho-physical unit. Mind and body cannot be separated.

So, if we reintegrate ourselves more often, we have fewer health problems and lead a life where we can enjoy good health and wellbeing.

How can you do this?

You can do this by being fully **RESPONSIBLE** for your whole self at all times, including those hours when you are 'at work'.

Having worked for a year as cabin crew for British Airways, I feel suitably qualified to use this analogy: In the pre-flight safety demonstration, cabin crew always say "Put **YOUR OWN** oxygen mask on **BEFORE** helping others." And so in life you should

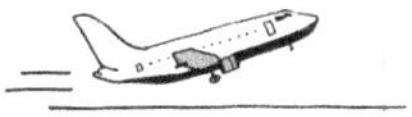

THINK OF YOURSELF FIRST BEFORE OTHERS!

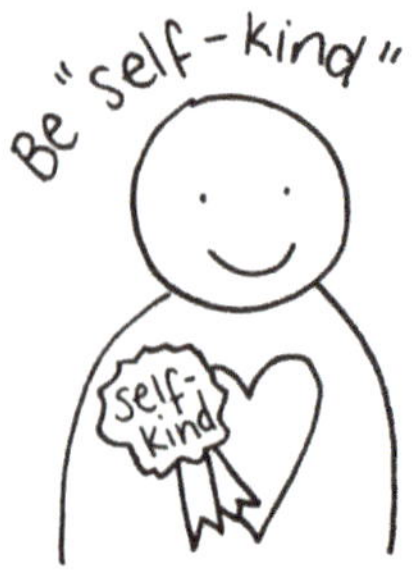

This is not selfishness but self care.

Unfortunately, in our society this ethos has been drummed out of us. We are almost too keen to give our power away nowadays.

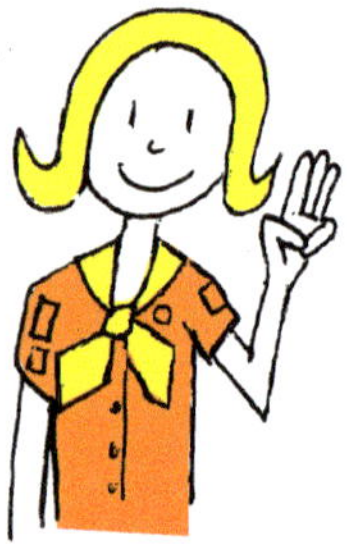

I remember saying "think of yourself first, before others" to my youngest daughter when she was around seven years old. She looked at me incredulously and said, "I thought you said you were a Brownie Guide." I replied that I was, at which she shook her head and said, "Well you don't know the Brownie Guide law then!" For those who similarly don't know, it is:
A Brownie Guide thinks of others before herself and does a good turn every day.

So, it struck me that our society starts shaping our beliefs very early on, encouraging us into putting ourselves last – but the cost of that is to ourselves. The consequences can be detrimental to our health and wellbeing and could spread out to our nearest and dearest and all of those around us in a negative way.

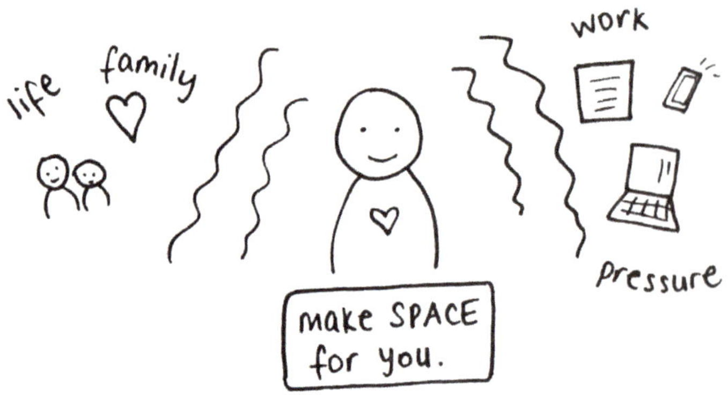

Therefore, I encourage you to say **"NO"** to that way of thinking and make some space for yourself in the centre of your busy life – even 'at work' or maybe especially 'at work'.

When you can practise this as a default 'attitude' to life, you can then be happier too – not overburdened or overwhelmed because **YOU ARE BEING RESPONSIBLE TO YOURSELF** first!

WHO IS THE MOST IMPORTANT PERSON IN YOUR LIFE?

Answer = YOU!

Now to start being 'self-kind' ('selfish' has negative connotations in our society so I encourage you to consider this way of being as 'self-kind' as a more positive way of thinking about it).

Familiar workplace issues

Do any of these sound like a 'fit' for you currently?

Do you suffer regularly with

- aches and pains?
- shoulder pain?
- back pain?
- neck pain?

Does it interfere frequently with your work/private life/passion/hobbies?

Are you

- frustrated that you can't do what you'd like to be able to do?
- feeling that life is unfair?

Would you like to

- be free to be yourself?
- embody your true hopes and desires?
- lead a fulfilling and rewarding life?
- be energised?
- be filled again with a childlike joy?
- be pain free and active with energy for hobbies?

Then read on to learn how to take care of yourself while you are at work, so you are able to enjoy your private life fully.

Desk/workstation set up

Here, I will address some common work situations and how we can manage ourselves better in our work environment.

THAT'S A TRUE WORK/LIFE BALANCE

In the words of the famous song from the musical Oliver:

CONSIDER YOURSELF

The Alexander Technique teaches us how to use our body well.

> The best ergonomic design will do nothing to prevent RSI if we are using ourselves badly. And if we are using ourselves well, we can function without undue strain even in difficult, awkward situations. Ergonomic solutions are not without value, but they are only a small part of the solution.
>
> **Robert Rickover**
> **on Ergonomics and RSI**

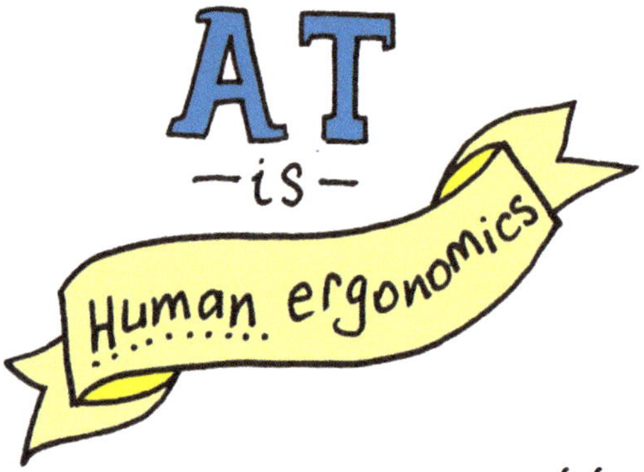

That said, desk height is important, as is the height of your chair. I'm going to give you a simple overview of some alternative ways of making yourself comfortable so you can work with ease.

Make sure your feet are fully in contact with the floor. Your seat bones need to be positively contacting the chair. Allow the ground and the chair to **FULLY** support you. If necessary, move to the front of your chair to have full foot contact with the ground. Or, if possible, put a yoga block underneath your feet so you can have your back **AND** your feet fully supported at the same time. Accept and receive all the support you can from the environment you are working in: this enables you to give more to your work because you are fully supported! See? It makes absolute sense to pay attention to **HOW** you are set up in order to work!

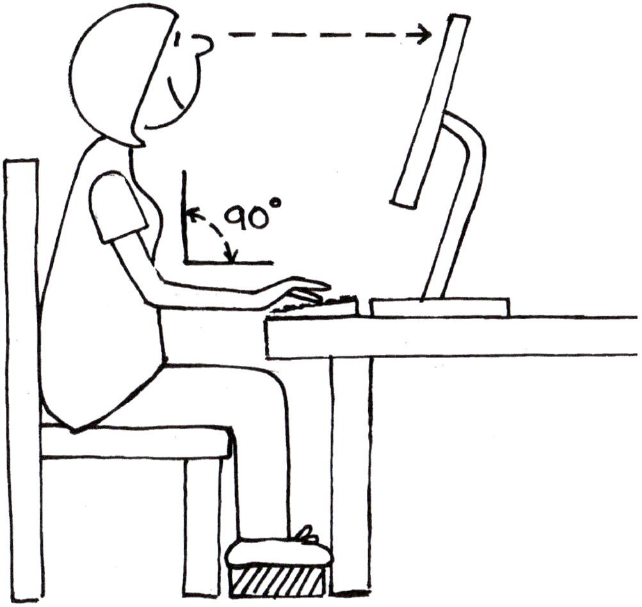

A great seat to work with is the **Wavestool**. Check it out as a great way to stay supported and flexible while you work. It also affords a lot of freedom of movement in the torso – encouraging active body movement keeps the mind alive, too.

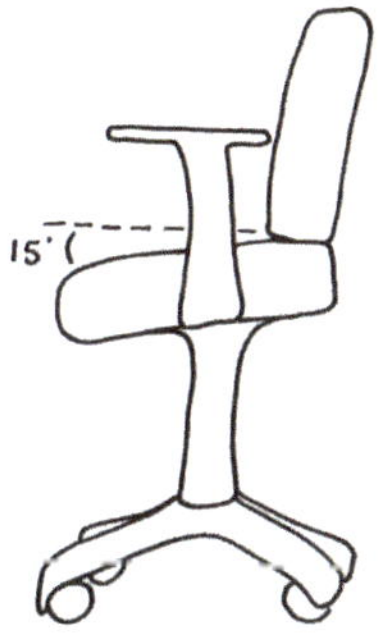

A 15 degree angle in your seat is great. Hips like it if they are higher than the knees

HIP, HIP HOORAY!

DON'T SLUMP

SUPPORT YOUR BACK,
then it can support you

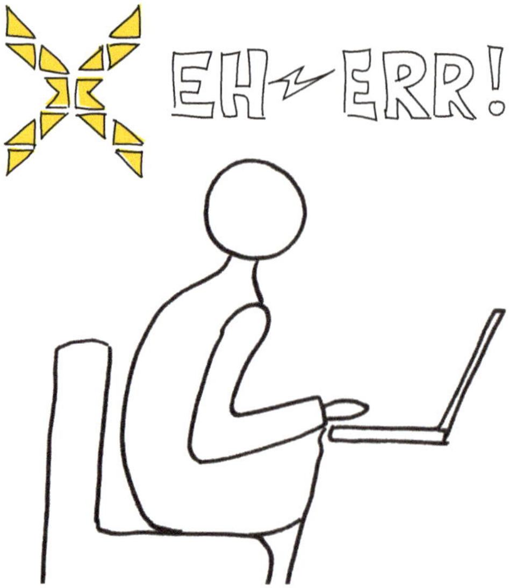

How are you sitting?

Let the seat bones take the full weight of your torso. Allow your vertebrae to organise themselves into their own natural curves.

Keep your back **BACK**. Beware of tipping or tilting the pelvis. Allow your spine to be **LONG**.

A LONG SPINE IS A STRONG SPINE

Direct the top of your spine to the ceiling above you and the base of your spine to the ground below you. Let your tummy out.

BREATHE!

Check if you are holding your breath.

Allow your head to move forwards and away from the top joint (the atlanto-occipital joint, where your head meets your spine).

MIND THE GAP!

If you need to move forwards, **PIVOT** from your hips to bring your whole torso closer to your screen or desk. Remember **THE HEAD LEADS** and the **BODY FOLLOWS.**

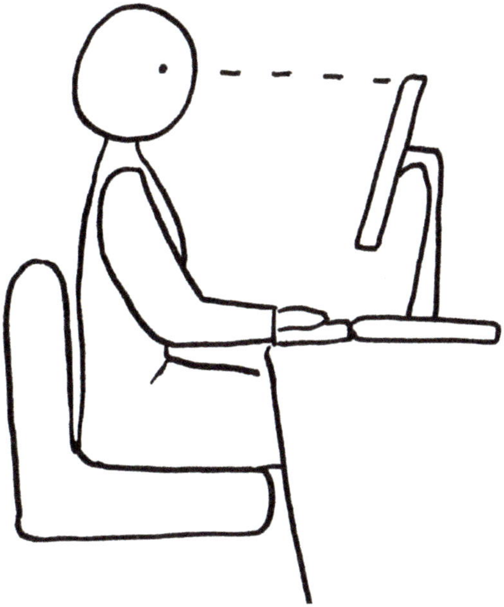

The height of the desk ideally allows your elbows to be at right angles or an obtuse angle; an acute angle is best avoided. Forearms should be parallel with the top of the desk.

Don't forget that your eyes can also move up and down independently of your head. Allow your eyes to receive information. Soften your eyes. Blink every 2-3 seconds. Avoid staring.

The top of your computer screen should be level with your eye line. Keeping your atlanto-occipital joint available really helps the eyes and neck to be freely available to you and flexible.

Allow your shoulder girdle to gently rest on top of your rib cage.

Remember these shoulder **DON'TS:**

NOT up

NOT down

NOT forwards

NOT back

What then?

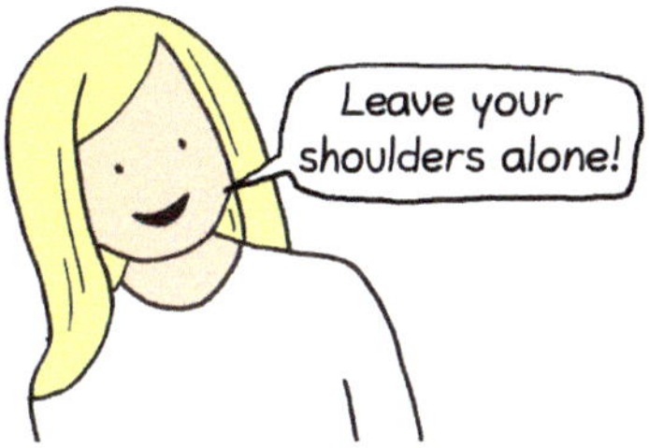

Shoulders flow one away from the other. Human arms in nature hang freely alongside the torso. Check where yours are and then allow them to return 'home'.

DON'T STICK YOUR NECK OUT

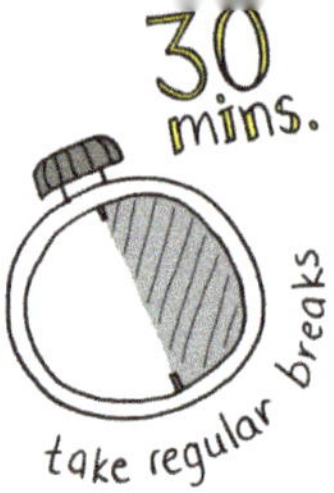

Have loose and bent elbows.

After 30 minutes, take a break.

Get up and walk around, blink, breathe and have some water.

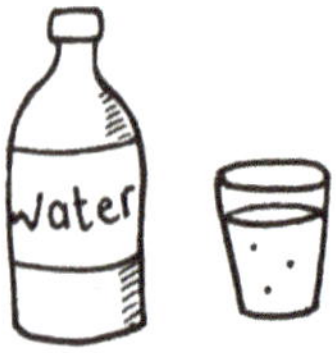

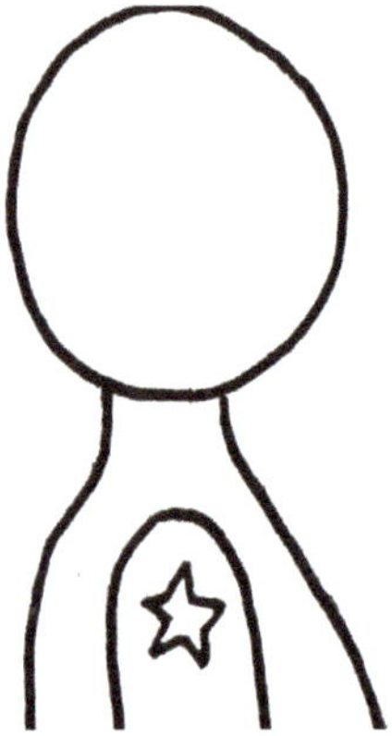

☆ shoulders hang freely
☆ check where yours are
☆ allow them to return 'home'

DON'T HOLD YOUR BREATH! Sometimes we do this unconsciously when we are concentrating or listening. It is possible to do both of these **AND** breathe; in fact it's beneficial if we can continue freely allowing the breath into and out of our systems while working. Are you doing this?

Pay attention to **YOU** while you work.

Mindful practice at your desk is possible and makes you more available to yourself and others.

Laptop tips

Continuing with the Oliver theme we can:

REVIEW THE SITUATION!

IT AIN'T WHAT YOU DO IT'S THE WAY THAT YOU DO IT ... remember?

So **HOW** can we use ourselves well when using a laptop?

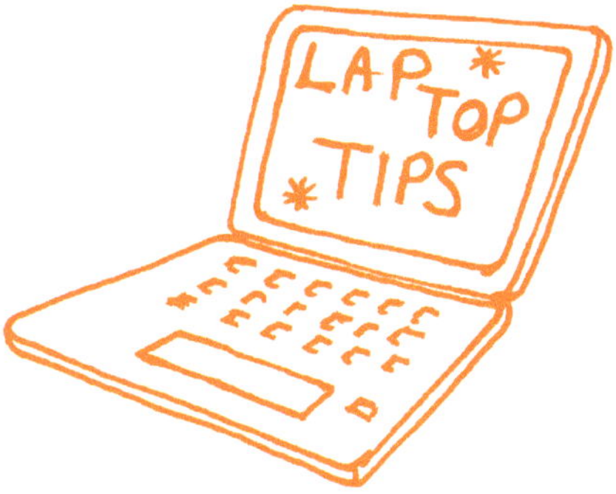

If you are at a table or desk, you can apply thought to **HOW** you are sitting.

Again, make sure your feet are **FULLY** contacting the ground. Are your seat bones making positive contact with the chair you are sitting on? Give the appropriate time to ensure that this **IS** happening **RIGHT NOW**. Allow your entire spinal column to come into natural alignment: top of the spine flowing directly up to the ceiling; base of your spine flowing directly towards the ground below you. Support your back. Allow your head to flow away from the top of the spine.

Allow the eyes to softly float down if you need to read something at the lower end of your screen.

There's always a trade off with a laptop but, as long as you are being mindful and

☆ Soften your eyes

☆ allow them to receive information

☆ avoid staring

paying full, undivided attention to yourself during the process, you should be able to manage the conditions well.

If you like the keyboard flat to the table top, your eyes and head will need to be freely available to scan the lower and outer edges of the screen. If this is not comfortable or possible, **RAISE** the laptop slightly onto a yoga block or a thick hardback book. The compromise here is that your keyboard is then higher up. Keep your elbows soft and allow your hands to lengthen away from the elbows. Think width and space to wrists and whole forearm. **DON'T TIGHTEN.**

Remember, your arms begin at the base of your spine. Are you truly taking this fact into consideration and applying it to your actual practice of using the keyboard in this position?

BREATHE, blink and set a timer to remind you to take a break after 30 minutes.

If possible, go for a walk outside, get some **FRESH** air and a change into a more natural scenery!

Thinking and learning involve the **WHOLE BODY, NOT JUST THE HEAD!** Often we're too 'in our heads'.

Vision on

To keep your peripheral vision alive when you're online, **TRY THIS:**

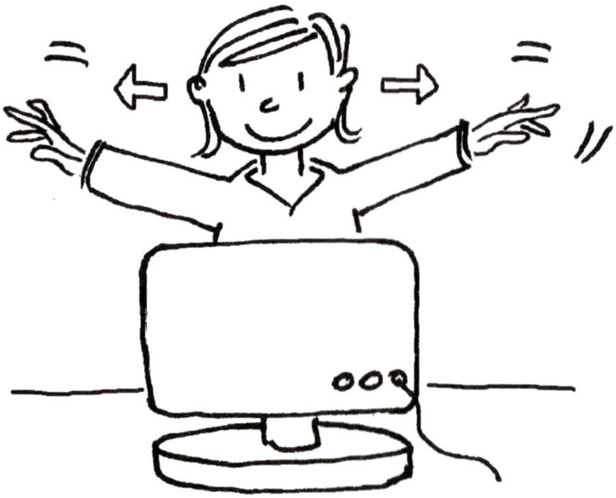

- Once an hour, wiggle your fingers either side of your eyes. Now send your arms backwards and notice at which point your hands go out of your line of sight.
- Shut your eyes for 30 seconds. Give them a rest. Computer screens are **SO** tiring for the eyes.
- Now try the wiggly fingers game again. Different isn't it? I'll bet your peripheral vision has improved!

Try looking into the distance, too, every 10 minutes. Doing that allows the lens to lengthen. There's not enough of that in our digital age when so much of our time involves an unnaturally brightly lit screen with many pixels for the eyes to accommodate.

Get outside into natural daylight as often as possible. Interaction with nature balances our rhythms and re-ignites our senses and, of course, is a **WHOLE BODY** experience.

If you can, keep a **LIVE** plant on your desk, something with texture, depth and height to keep alive your spatial awareness. Too much interaction with a flat screen encourages two-dimensional thinking! You need to return to a 3-D real world frequently to reintroduce balance to the visual system.

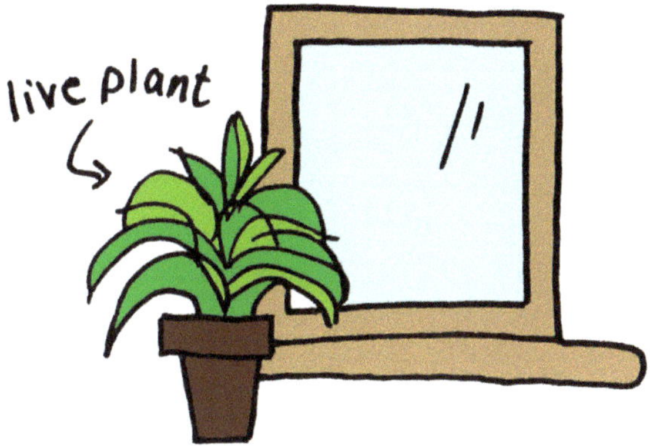

Can you be even more extravagant and introduce something with movement to your workspace? A goldfish is excellent or, better still, a pair of goldfish as their movement also helps to keep your attention alive!

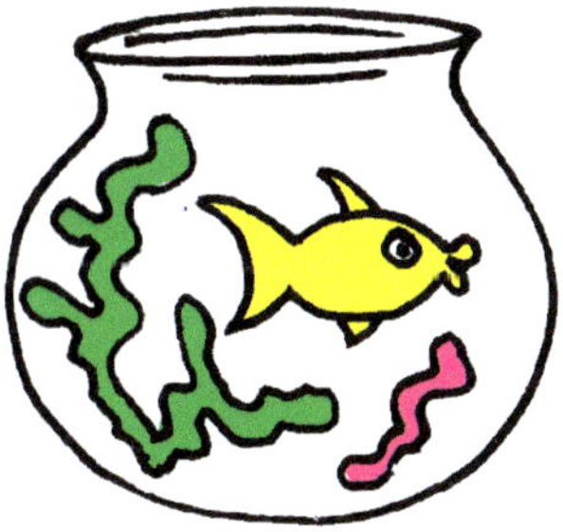

Colour delights the eyes and mind, so try to introduce it into the workplace – don't have it too sterile!

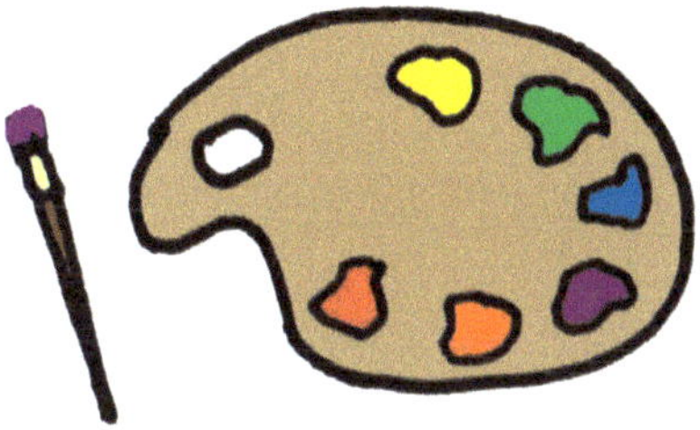

Well-lit space lessens eyestrain, but beware strip lighting, which is difficult for eyes due to the constant flicker. Don't make your eyes work too hard.

The eyes are just the vehicle: the **VISUAL CORTEX** is actually in the back of the brain. Allow time for visual information to go in **THROUGH** the eyes and then reach the visual cortex. That way, sense can be made of the information.

Vision is made up of imagination and memory. What are you **EXPECTING** to see? Notice instead what happens when you just allow your eyes to see what's **ACTUALLY** happening in front of them, with NO expectation, judgement or comment! You'll find it **MUCH** less of a strain!

Keep your desk clear and organised. A clear work space gives a clear mind!

Be mindful of your body temperature, too. Keep warm! This is particularly important if you work in an air-conditioned office. Then it is even more important to take regular breaks and try to get outside in daylight – in your lunch break or at some point in the day – to re-connect with nature.

“I always slumped in my office chair and over-reached to my keyboard but after several sessions with my Alexander Technique teacher it all became quite clear – good posture together with exercise will pay great rewards in later years. Yes I still do slump occasionally and don't use my sit bones but after a very short time I do remember and re-adjust myself. Once you understand the basic principles it is easy to follow!

Austin Reynolds – Keen Cyclist and Business Director”

CHAPTER SIX

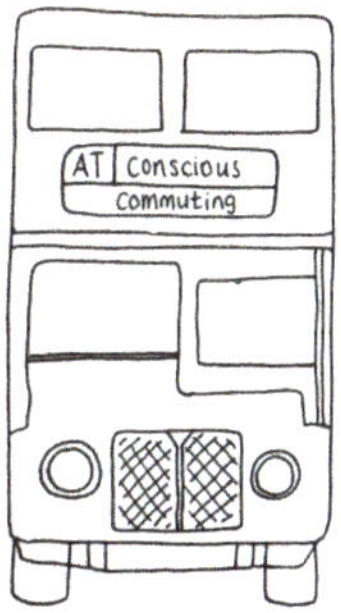

CONSCIOUS COMMUTING – PLANES, TRAINS AND AUTOMOBILES

I really love the film Planes, Trains and Automobiles starring Steve Martin. While it is reasonably old (it was released in 1987), it perfectly depicts the craziness we encounter in our modern lives. Rushing from place to place with hundreds of other similarly stressed and rushed human beings is commonplace!

So, how do we make space for ourselves if public transport and air travel are a regular or even daily part of our lives? It IS possible.

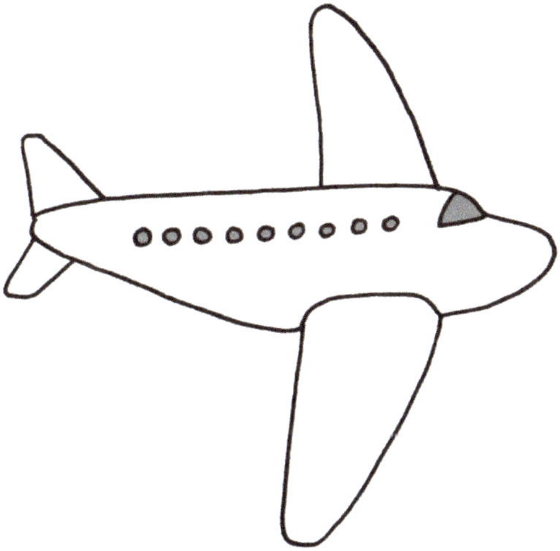

Planes

Plan your journey well. Do you know that saying "If you fail to plan, you plan to fail"? It applies here! Select appropriate flight times for your body rhythms, where possible. Pack ahead of time and go to bed early the night before so you're well rested.

TIME is a key factor. Allowing plenty of time to travel to the airport is worthwhile, as we all know travel is often unpredictable. Bring along healthy snacks and water and don't forget your flexible attitude!

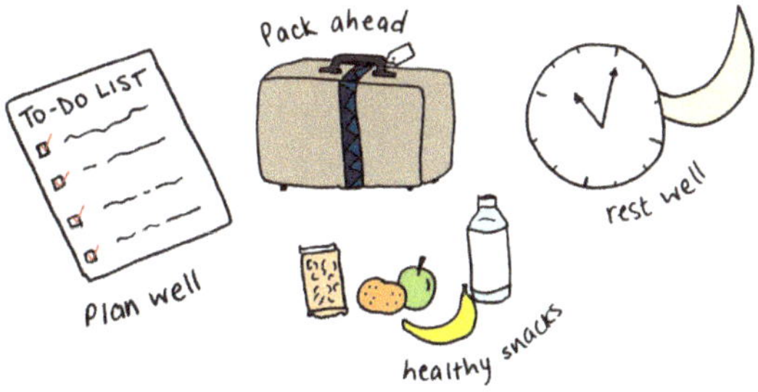

Allow plenty of time to negotiate your way through the airport, too. Plenty of time allows for a more relaxed integrated version of you. Crowds and queues are best negotiated with time on your side.

TIME PRESSURE = ANXIETY

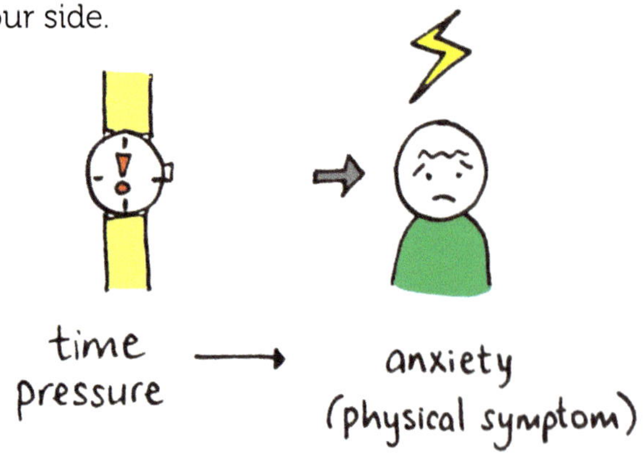

That will manifest in you physically and will be addressed more fully a little later in the book.

Breathe, take your time. Be with your self fully while you begin your journey through the airport. Checking in, going through security, perusing the shops or sitting in an airport lounge – whatever you're doing – keep all your senses alert and with you.

Tune in to yourself; make sure you are comfortable. Visit the toilet before boarding. These things may seem pretty obvious but **COMFORT IS KEY!**

CHOOSE COMFORT!

Consider a neck pillow plus a scarf or pashmina. They will keep you warm and comfortable on board.

As regards the airline seat: this depends on which class of travel you are in. They are never wide enough for my liking. In fact, they seem to get narrower as the years go by and I don't think my own girth has altered that much!

So, how can we maximise our comfort and arrive at our destination looking and feeling intact?

Wear comfortable, loose clothing and flat shoes. You can be smart and comfortable. Our bodies expand with the change in air pressure so allow for this to happen.

Restrictive clothing or shoes are not a good idea on a plane.

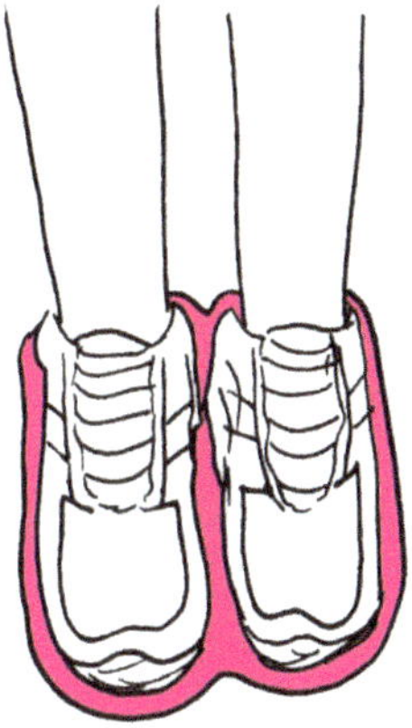

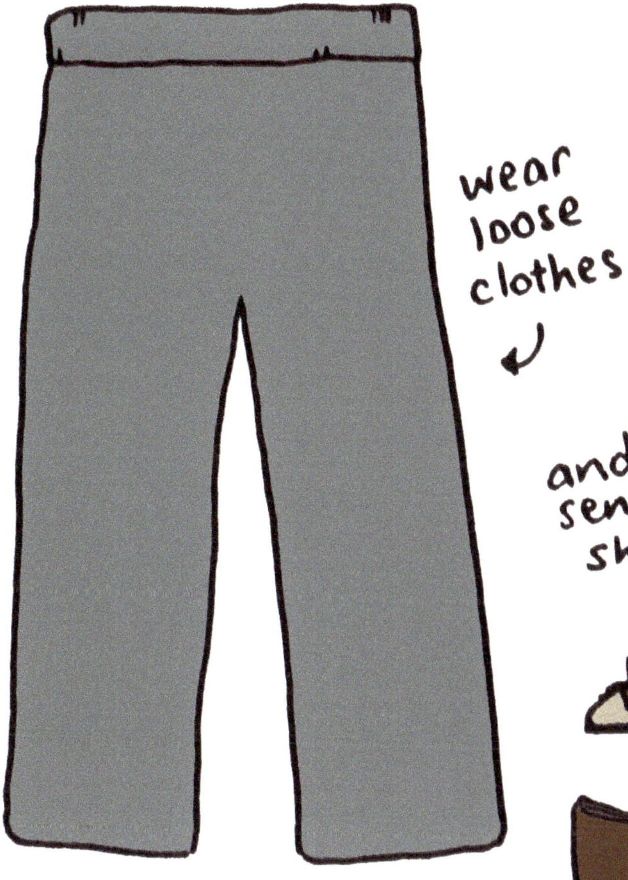

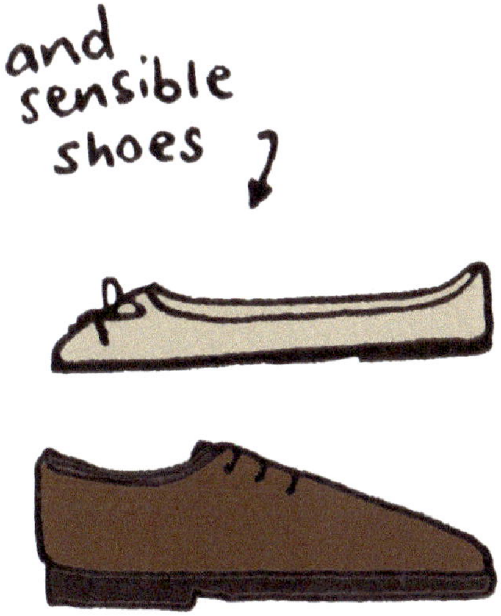

When you're in your seat, **CLAIM YOUR SPACE**.

Yes, you might be uncomfortably close to your neighbour but still claim **YOUR** space. Don't compromise yourself to spare your fellow passenger from space invasion! It's their business what they do with their body! Make it your business to look after yours as best you can.

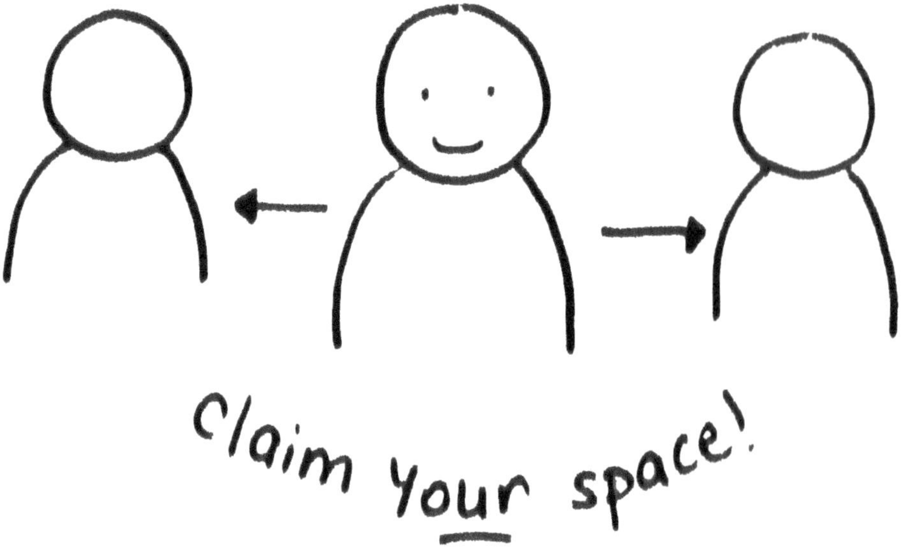

Make sure your feet are fully in contact with the ground.

Allow them to rest on the floor underneath the knees or split them one in front of the other.

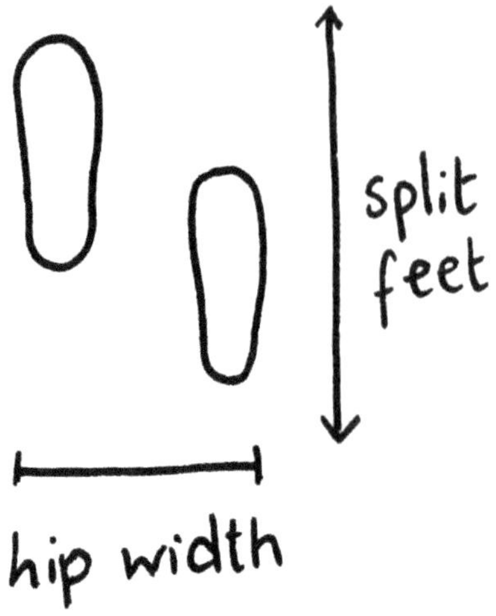

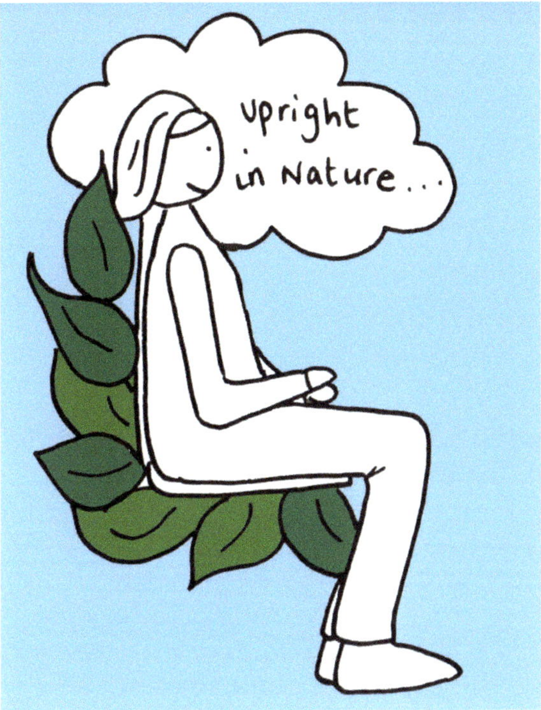

The important thing is that the lower leg supports the knee.

Find your seat bones, and really direct them to make contact with the airline seat. Sit back in your chair so that the back of your pelvis and your entire back are supported fully by the back of the seat. If there are any gaps, plug them with the airline's small pillow or roll a jumper into a ball.

Make sure you can feel the chair's support against the back of the pelvis, your whole spine and the back of your shoulders. Ideally, the back of your head should be supported, too.

Remember to direct your shoulders one away from the other, allowing the shoulder girdle to gently rest on the ribcage.

Remind yourself of the shoulder don'ts:

NOT up

NOT down

NOT forwards

NOT back

What then? **Nothing** – leave them alone!

Elbows should be heavy; wrists flowing away from the elbows; hands flowing away from the wrists.

If you worry about airborne infections from your fellow passengers, do consider a surgical mask. You can buy them in packs from your local pharmacy.

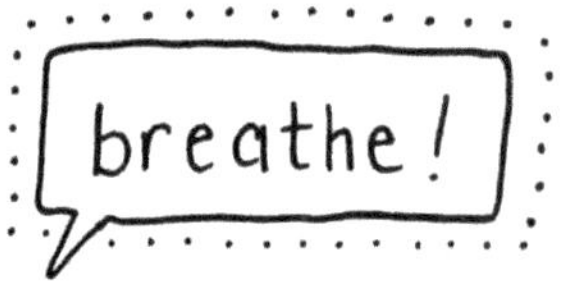

Allow your neck muscles to free up from any unnecessary tension. Your head should flow away from the top of your spine. Your whole spine should be able to lengthen and widen. Let your knees be soft and flowing out from free hips that are releasing out from the pelvis.

Your pelvis should be beautifully anchored to your seat. Use the armrests, if they're of an appropriate height for your upper arms. Elbows should be at right angles or an obtuse angle, with forearms fully accepting their support. If the armrests aren't at the right height, move them up and out of the way, and let your hands – palms up or down – rest on your thighs comfortably.

If airline noise concerns you, consider noise-cancelling headphones. Inflight entertainment usually includes some helpful tips on health and wellbeing in the air so do view those and follow the current advice.

Heed all the safety briefings first, too. However frequent a flyer you are, make sure you're au fait with the aircraft you are travelling on this time.

Count the seats forwards and back to your nearest exit: in an emergency you'll be glad of that information!

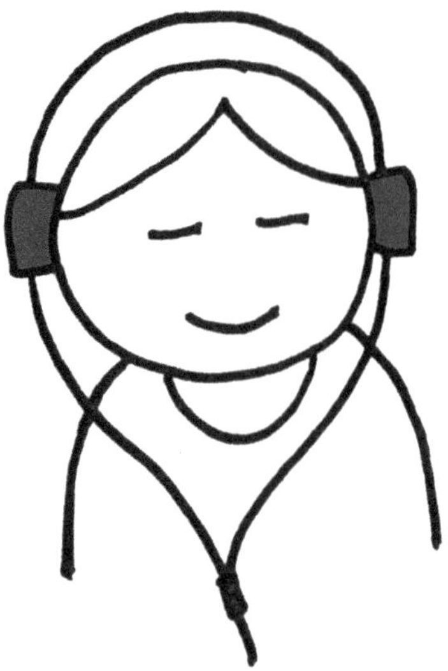

Remain hydrated during your flight. Drink some water or fruit juice every 20 minutes. Avoid alcohol. If the cabin crew don't bring drinks around frequently, ask them for some or drink your own.

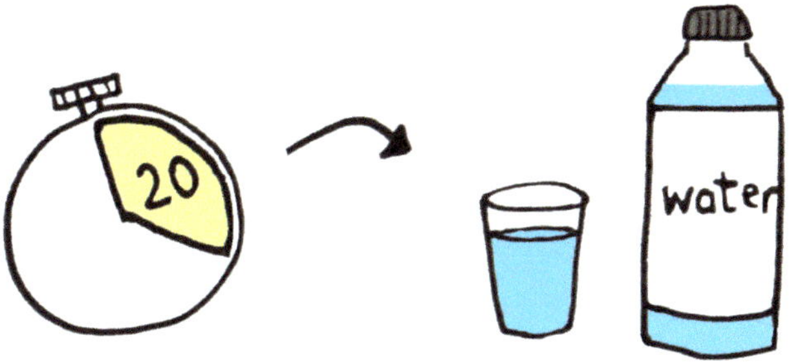

On a long flight it's advisable to get up and move around to mobilise yourself.

When you're in your seat, remember to keep on claiming **ALL** of your space. Don't collapse or tilt away from your neighbour. Your spine should be upright; your pelvis anchoring you to your seat; shoulders gently resting on the rib cage. Shoulders, hips and knees should flow away from each other.
Remember: **YOU come first!**

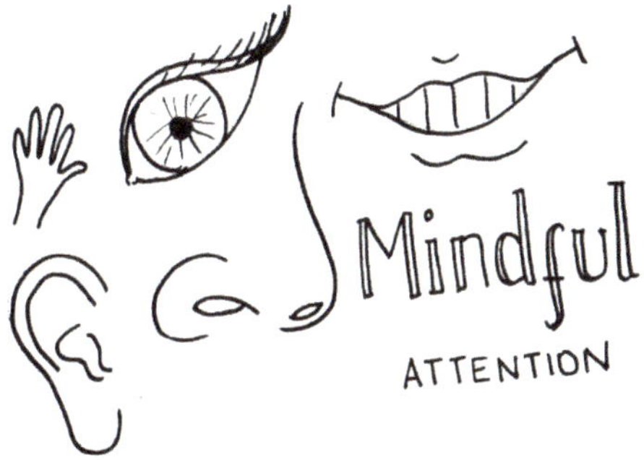

Practise your constructive rest in your seat. Listen to an audio version to mindfully rest your whole self.

Hopefully, you will arrive at your destination refreshed and relaxed!

After arrival, switch to local time as soon as possible and try to eat meals at local time to limit jet lag. Natural daylight helps, as does gentle exercise.

The **'Whispered Ah'** is a very effective restorative exercise for breathing. If you are having AT lessons, I recommend that you ask a teacher to show you this practice.

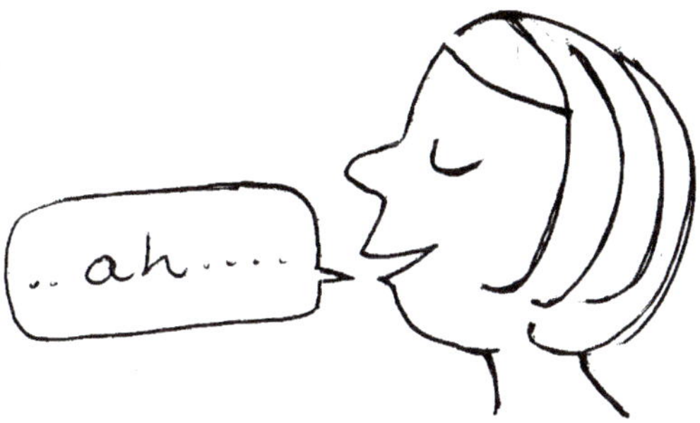

And, of course, semi-supine at your destination is very helpful to enable your body to recuperate from the effects of air travel.

I have found it easier than I originally thought to incorporate aspects of AT into my life. I work as cabin crew, doing long haul flights, so my life has little routine to it. However, there are definitely times where I now have my 'AT hat' on as part of my working day. Probably the easiest one to remember and one of the most beneficial is when I am doing 'Smiley Goodbyes' at the end of a flight. I think about my posture and make sure that my weight is evenly spaced between and on my feet; my arms are by my sides and relaxed; and that everything 'lines up' from my ankles to the top of my head.

It often takes 15 minutes or more to say goodbye when disembarking hundreds of passengers from a 747 and there isn't another time when I would be solely just standing and can give focus to my practice. It also has the added benefit that the posture looks good. As crew, we have to be aware not to have closed body language when engaging with customers and it is easy at the end of a long flight to lean against a bulkhead or cross your arms. AT teaches a way of standing and moving that creates open body language, which looks approachable and welcoming to others.

Natalie Proud – Virgin Atlantic Stewardess

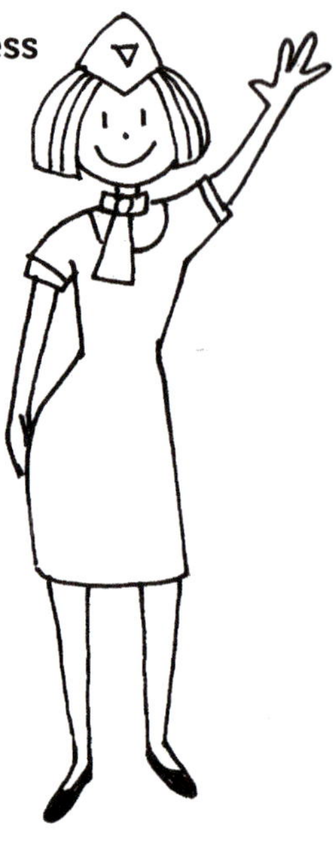

Trains

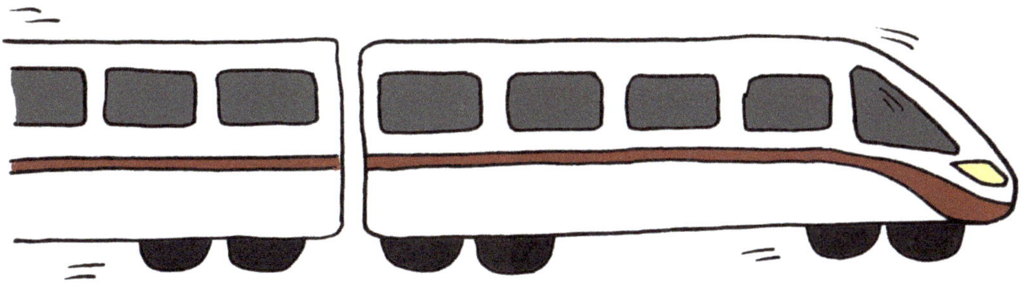

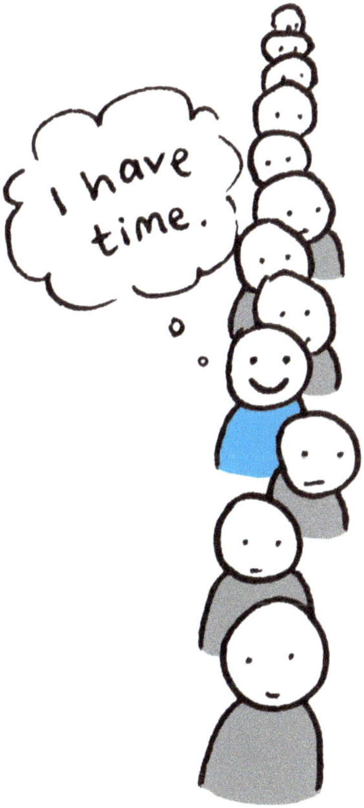

Many of us commute to work daily using overground and underground trains. The secret to a carefree commute is allowing the actual time you need to complete your journey from A to B. The journey starts before you leave your front door.

Set your alarm early enough so that you have the chance to rise, shower and eat breakfast, and are therefore nourished and equipped to face the day. Set aside enough time to reach the train station.

Travel is unpredictable; squeezing your time gives no margin for delays, cancelled trains and so on, which results in anxiety in **YOU**. This anxiety can be avoided by allowing for events to change, thus making for a calmer less stressed 'you'.

Buying your ticket ahead in a less hurried atmosphere is also a wise move. There is nothing more frustrating than a slow-moving queue when you're under time pressure to get somewhere.

As for the train/Tube journey itself: keep all your senses alive and with you. If there are no seats and you have to stand, that will be fine if you pay some mindful attention as to **HOW** you are standing in the moving carriage.

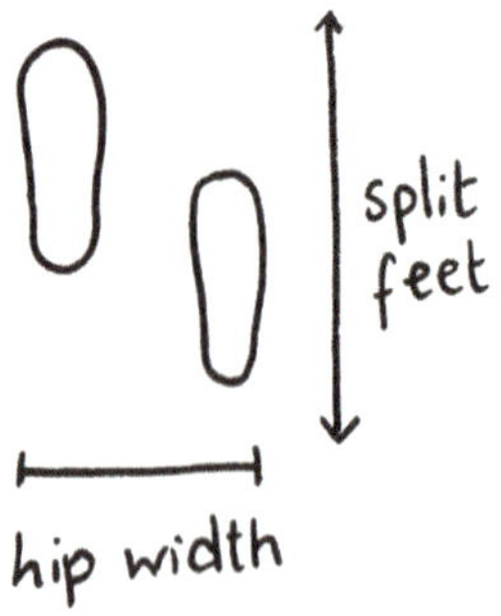

Stand with feet hip-width apart. Split feet (i.e. one foot ahead of the other) give you a wide and more balanced stance and a more stable base to commute comfortably from.

As before, plug in your feet, ground yourself and allow your springy feet to accept the full support of the floor. Keep your three natural hinges in the leg **FREE**: these are the ankles, knees and hips.

By doing this, you give your legs the opportunity to support your torso flexibly and you will be able to **WITHSTAND** (very appropriate word!) the train's movement. The pelvis should be heavy, anchoring the lower end of your torso and spine. Your shoulder girdle should gently rest on the ribcage. Give your ribs full permission to move fully and freely with respiration; your sternum (breastbone) floating. Your spine should be suspended from the head, which is free to fall up and forwards, away from the atlanto-occipital joint.

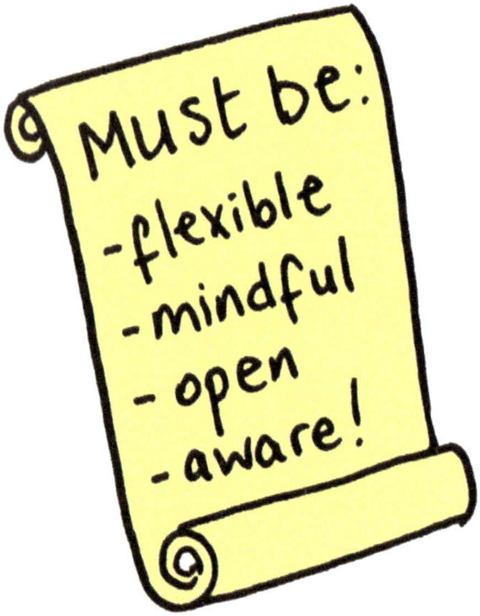

The jaw should hang from the skull freely; teeth lightly contacting each other. Shoulders, hips and knees should be away from each other. If you need to hang on to an overhanging strap or rail, make sure your arms are releasing out of your lengthening back.

Stand your ground, claim your space fully with confidence and be open and flexible to the journey. Respect your personal space and keep it fairly close to yourself, appropriate to the number of passengers you are sharing the space with. In this way, you should be able to reach your destination reasonably unscathed, having been flexible, mindful, open and aware.

Automobiles

Cars are very much part of our modern lives. How to set up your driving position is an essential part of this process of looking after yourself. Some of us sit for hours every week in our cars. Follow this advice and driving can become a pleasure again – especially when you arrive at your destination feeling full of vitality and in no discomfort.

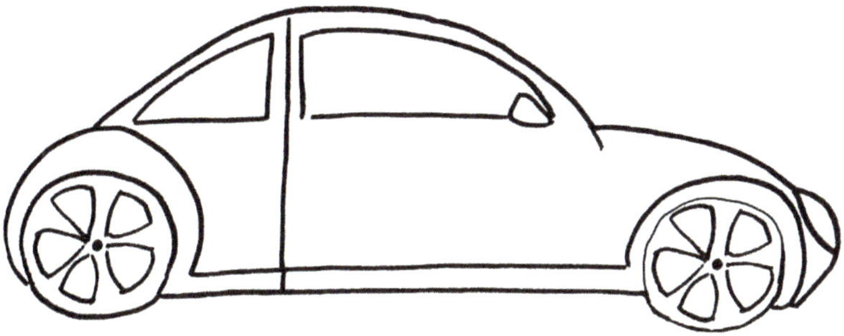

Car seats are poorly designed. In a way, they reflect our poor posture! They encourage the shoulders forwards.

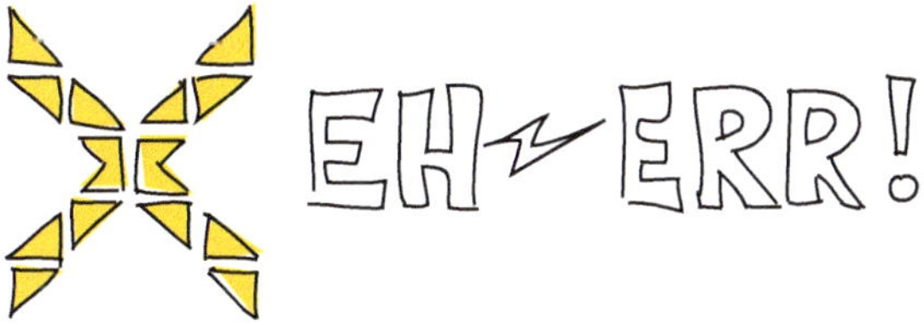

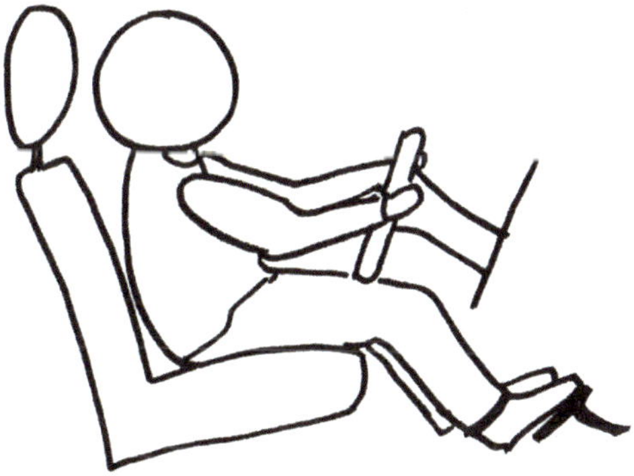

But we can make the best out of a bad situation.
Put the seat-back upright. No 'cool' leaning back, please!

When sitting, the torso is upright in nature. When we are driving we are sitting,
so ensure you set up your driving conditions so that your torso can be upright.
Most people have the seat-back tilted backwards.
Make the seat base flat,
if possible.

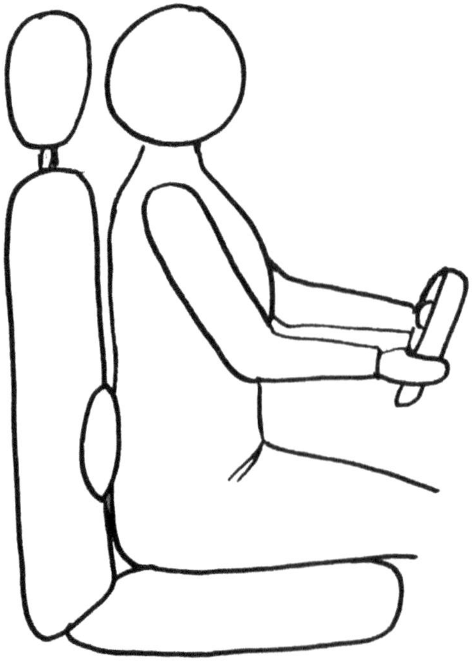

This helps you to connect your seat bones to the car seat and allows your pelvis to support your spine and the lower end of your torso. Remember, your vertebrae can organise themselves into their perfectly natural curves, stacking up one on top of another.

Direct your tailbone to the floor.
Direct the top of your spine to the roof of your car. Allow your head to fall up and forwards, away from the top of your spine.
The jaw lends its weight to the front aspect of your skull.

Let the seat back fully support your spine. It can be useful to have a small bolster pillow, a CD case or an A-Z to place between the shoulder blades. It helps to give a reference point to the thoracic spine, making it less likely to collapse. Move the whole seat forwards or back to accommodate the length of your legs to the pedals, with knees soft and available.

Now move your rear view mirror. This is your standard. If you can't see into it, check how you are sitting before you alter it! The headrest in line with the seat back is another useful contact point for the back of the head. If the headrest encourages your neck forwards, move your whole body forwards and fill the gap with a firm, supportive bolster.

Keep your shoulders open. Collar bones should be long, shoulder blades floating home on the back of the ribcage, allowing the armpits to be spacious – not clenched tight to the torso. Elbows should be heavy: your steering wheel is a useful contact for the arms to lengthen away from. Don't grip the steering wheel too hard. A gentle curling of the fingers, coming out of arms that begin at the base of the spine, with soft elbows, is a helpful way of driving without stress.

I like driving in my car ... goes the song from Madness. Now you can too!

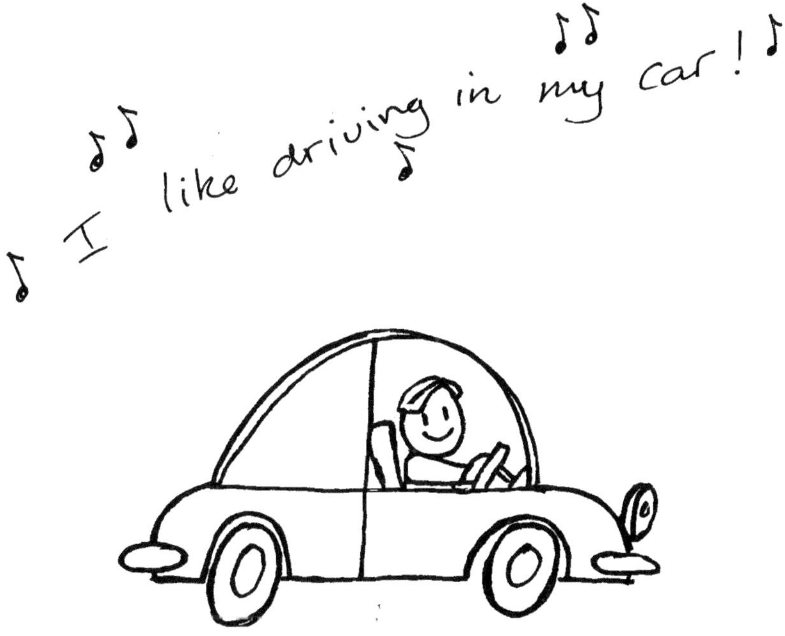

HOW TO MONKEY AROUND

- THINKING IN ACTIVITY

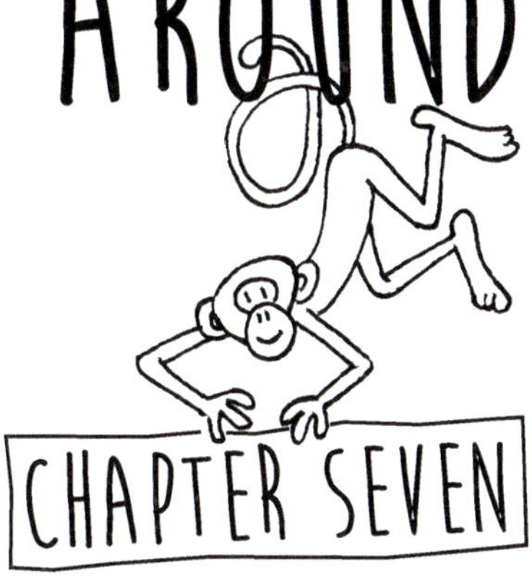

1. **Do you wish your daily chores were easier to manage physically?**
2. **Do you have a hobby you love or used to love but no longer have the energy to manage fully?**
3. **Are there some daily activities that seem like 'hard work' to you right now?**

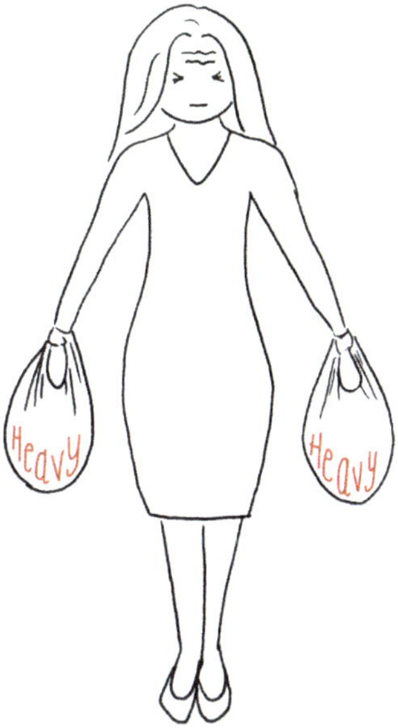

If you answered **YES** to any of the above questions, I can relate very well to where you are 'at'. I vividly remember wishing it was easier to dry my hair!

My hair dryer had become impossibly heavy for me to manage at the peak of my repetitive strain injury. I had similar thoughts about driving, picking up my children, lifting heavy bags, carrying my handbag on my 'favourite shoulder' and baking (beating a mixture by hand was too difficult).

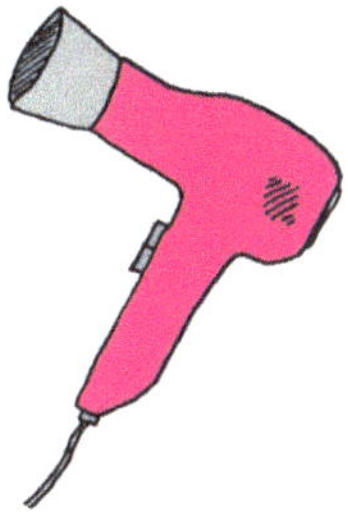

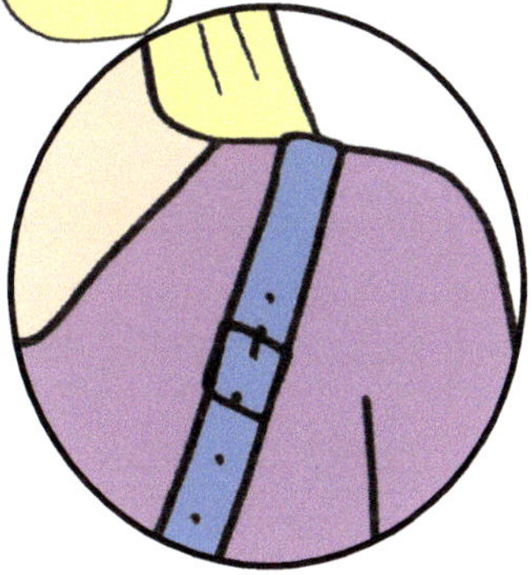

Certain gym exercises were unattainable by me.
For example: side plank on my right hand side was not possible for a while.

And handwriting was truly very painful.

BUT ... guess what! **NOT ANY MORE.** Why not? Because I practise Alexander Technique **EVERY DAY**. I apply it to all of my daily activities so that my habits do not take the reins in my body.

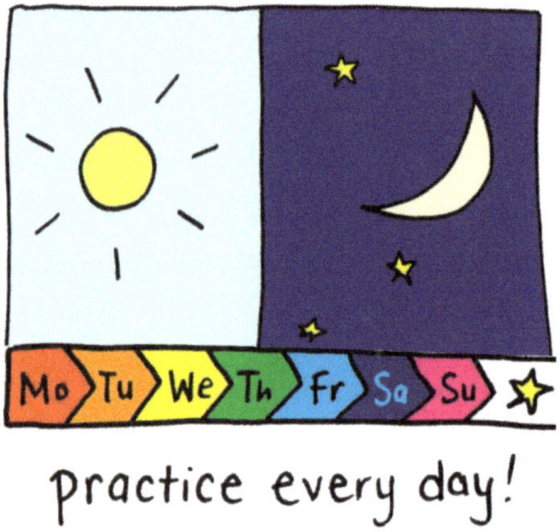
Mo Tu We Th Fr Sa Su
practice every day!

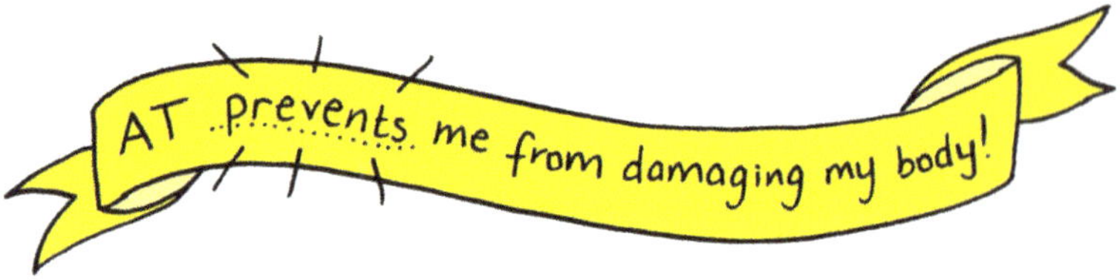
AT prevents me from damaging my body!

HOW can Alexander Technique do this?

It's all in the mind ... in the thinking.

> I came to the Alexander Technique with a very specific injury, which I planned to fix. I did not realise that I had stumbled upon a whole new way of being and moving: a technique ideally suited to helping us cope with the demands of life in the twenty-first century, and one that offers prevention of pain as well as a cure. As such, awareness of and access to the Alexander Technique ought to be widespread.
>
> **Roberta Wolff – Pianist**

Before you begin any activity, chore or hobby: **STOP**.

This momentary pause allows you the time to choose an appropriate reaction, response or plan of action using conscious direction of your whole self.

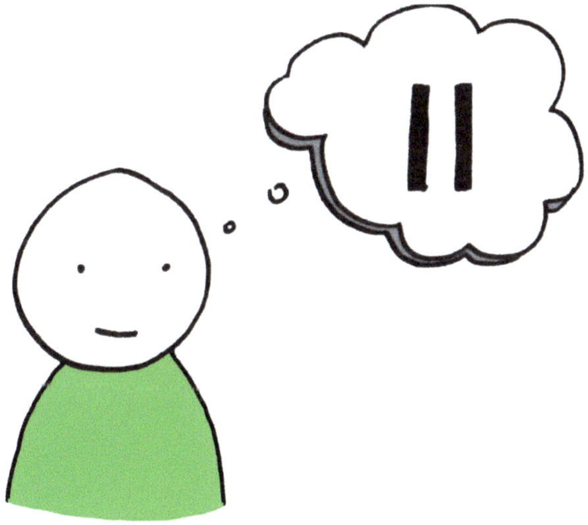

Eh?

Alexander called it **INHIBITION**. Let me explain ...

Before I had heard of the Alexander Technique I was a **REACTIVE** person. Using a simple example I will demonstrate the way I was responding to life at that time ...

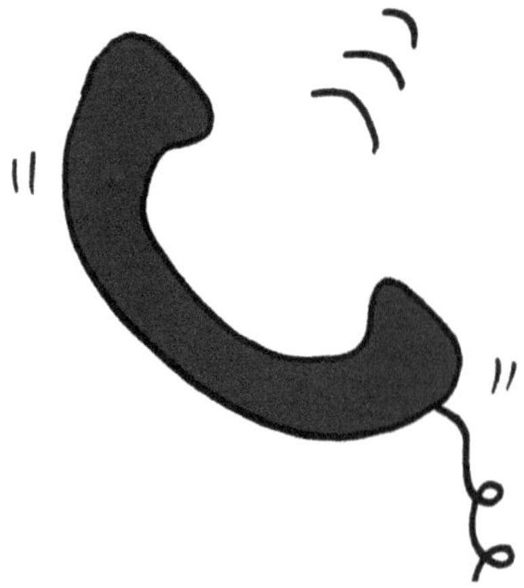

If the telephone rang, whatever I was doing, I would drop everything, **RUSH** to answer it **BEFORE** the second ring, **HOLDING MY BREATH** during the whole process, running across the room to pick up the handset and 'beat the clock'.

It seems almost funny to me now! You get an insight though into where I was 'at' and, as you can imagine, this way of being was not serving me very well at all. It affected me physically in the form of a repetitive strain injury. I was stopped in my tracks. My body could not continue that way of being used any longer.

SOMETHING HAD TO CHANGE!

That something was **ME**! And my approach to life.

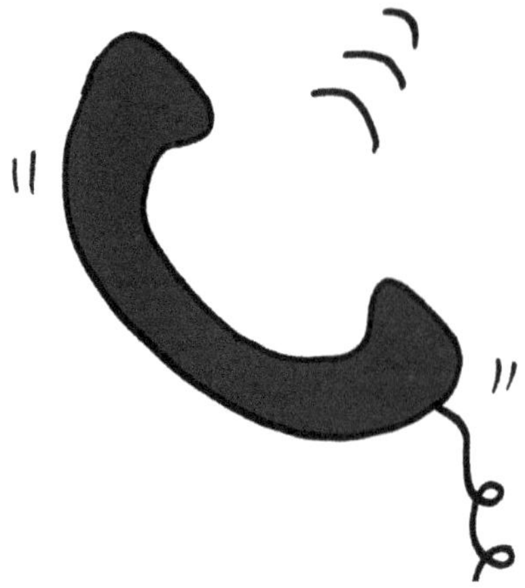

So now knowing the Alexander Technique, my approach to life is **VERY** different, and one that is a whole lot more balanced and healthy as a result.

To go back to the telephone situation again...How do I respond to that now?

Ask for quiet

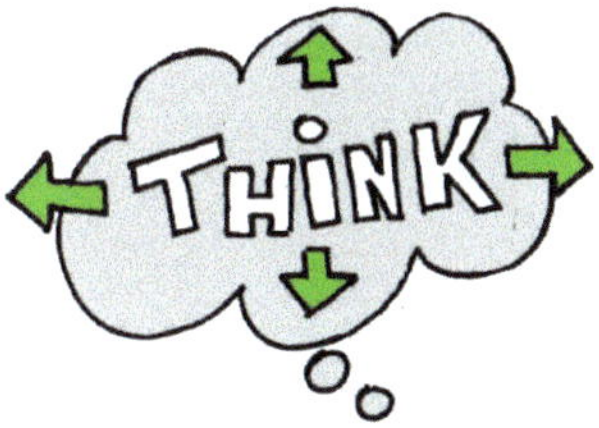

Through your directions

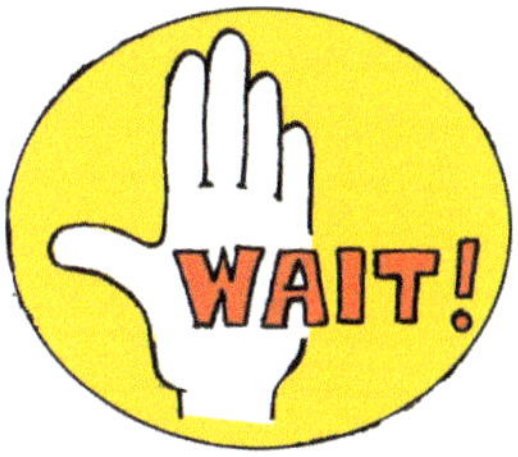

For freedom to appear

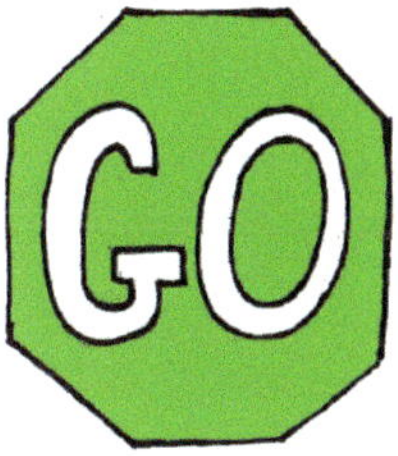

Move freely and with ease

Let's set the scene: I'm in the kitchen cooking and the phone rings. I hear it and **think...stop!**

I then send my **FOUR ALEXANDER DIRECTIONS** to myself:

1. **Let the neck be free** so that...
2. **The head can go forwards and up** in order that...
3. **The whole spine can lengthen and the whole back can widen** and...
4. **The knees can go forwards and away**

In addition, I make sure I am **BREATHING**.

I wait for freedom to appear, then I **MOVE** freely and with ease to pick up the phone handset, probably between the second and third ring – in a **MUCH BETTER STATE** than my 'un-Alexandered' self did!

I can also think more clearly, speak coherently, listen intently and it's a much calmer, mindful process all round.

Being able to pay attention to yourself in this way has huge benefits, not only to you but also to those around you. Your whole being functions much more efficiently and smoothly in this way.

And you have fewer adrenaline rushes!

This mental process can be applied any time, any place, anywhere. It's a discrete aid to your self and your mind. Alexander's helpful directions taken on board and utilised in your daily activities, whatever they may be!

Monkey

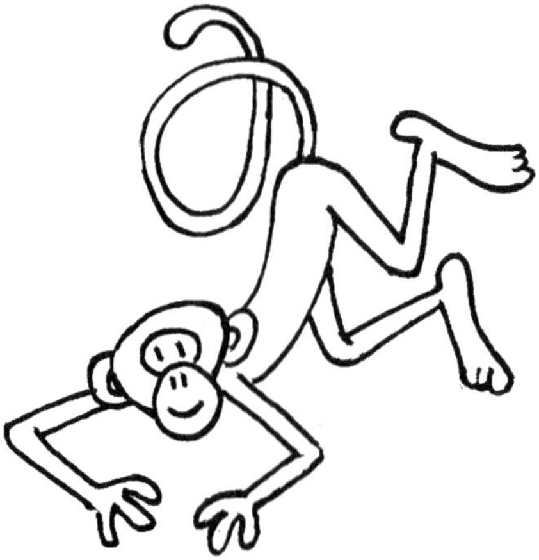

This is a term we use in the Alexander Technique. It's as it sounds and is a position of **'mechanical advantage'** for the body.

Where have you heard that expression before? Yes, in this book (see Chapter 4)!

Going into the chair from standing, as described earlier in the book, can be considered to be a **bunch of monkeys**.

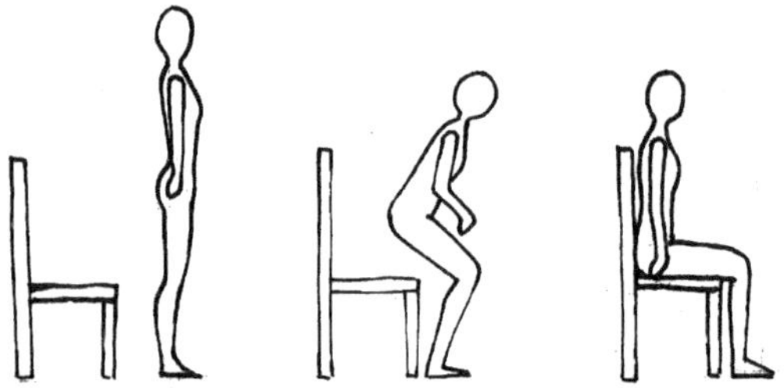

In essence, the spine is long, the head is free from the top of the spine, the torso in one whole piece and the hips, knees and ankles are free to facilitate fluid, easy movement, recruiting the deep postural muscles of the back.

Alexander Technique semi-supine can be considered to be a **HORIZONTAL MONKEY**.

This is a reason why the practice is so beneficial. The whole system gets a restful opportunity to be reminded of this position of mechanical advantage.

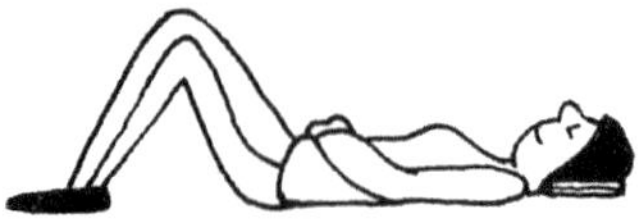

The body is fully supported; the entire spinal column revitalised and energised. Limbs are freed up; muscular knots undone. Helpful neural pathways are re-established to rediscover the way we 'used' our bodies before, as babies and toddlers.

If you have any small people in your life, children of your own, nephews, nieces, grandchildren, friends, neighbours ...
WATCH AND LEARN!

They will be using themselves in this way, mechanically advantageous to their surroundings. It's beautiful to watch: **SO** easy, **SO** graceful, **SO** fluid and **SO** full of life and vitality.

You still have the same latent ability in you.

Simply re-learning how to sit, stand, rest and move with ease is what this work is about.

AND the additional bonus is this:

When you understand your body and use it as nature intended

THE SKY IS THE LIMIT!

When we free up our physical selves, we free up our mental state, too.

Why?

We are one psycho-physical unit (more on that later).

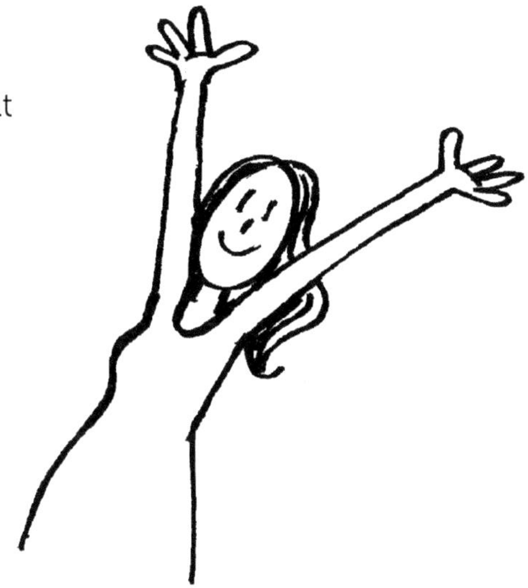

So, **what is Monkey** and how do we bring this into our lives?

This helpful advantageous stance is available to us whenever we are 'directing' our whole body.

Plug in your feet, receive the full support of the floor, think up off your ankles, up your calves, including the outer edges to your knees. Allow the knee caps to fall out from free hips; allow the knee joint to bend from the back through to the front, so it's 'on the latch' and the knees are forwards and flowing one away from the other.

The hip sockets release the legs away from the pelvis. Remember how far away from your brain your hips are!

Keep your spine long. Direct your tailbone to the ground below you. Allow the spine to organise itself into its natural curved uprightness, each vertebra 'stacking up' one on top of the other until the top of the spine flows directly up to the ceiling/sky above you.

Now let your head move delicately up away from the top joint and allow gravity to gently pull it forwards. Leave your spine alone and allow the jaw to lend its weight to the front of your skull.

BREATHE!

Allow your head to lead this movement; think up off free hips in order that the whole torso can angle forwards. Hinge from your hips now, sending your knees forwards.

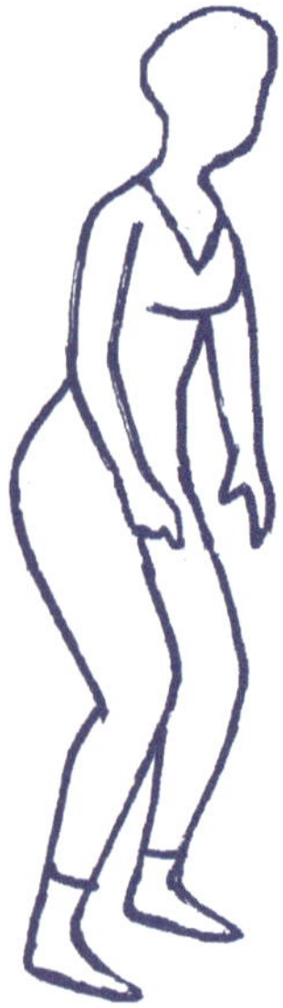

Allow your shoulders to flow one away from the other. Remember your shoulder don'ts

NOT up
NOT down
NOT forwards
NOT back

...just left alone

When you leave your whole body alone, freeing up your joints, your whole self is available for movement.

MONKEY = AVAILABLE YOU

Recruiting the deep postural muscles of the back is such a good idea! They contain more red muscle fibre within so they don't tire easily, like the muscles of the heart and diaphragm. Consider them your first-class levers.

The whole muscular 'suit' is then optimally primed and engaged, making for a super-efficient version of you, in other words 'natural'.

Think how often this **'monkey'** could be used. Anywhere! OK, here are some examples: pushing a supermarket trolley, pushing a buggy, washing up, driving, at work, at a computer screen, mowing the lawn, cycling, hiking, walking, horse riding, gardening, rowing, running, meditating, commuting, in the gym.

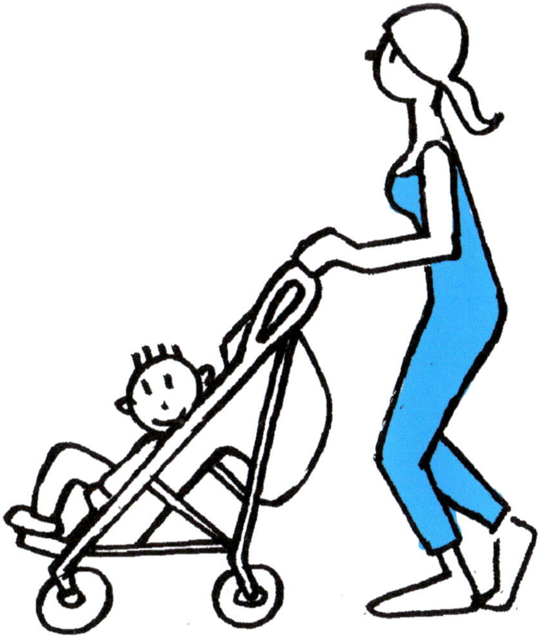

Get creative – I'm sure you can think of many more!

Be gentle with yourself. It can be quite a workout to begin with when you re-introduce this way of using your body in movement and activity. It may well take some time before the body can accommodate it again fully.

And my strong advice to you is to undertake some AT lessons to explore the concept fully. It is possible to misunderstand and, hey, sometimes what we think we're doing is **NOT** what we're **ACTUALLY** doing. We have, as Alexander says, 'faulty sensory appreciation'.

Alexander Technique retrains our distorted kinaesthetic awareness but it takes time.

Hands-on guidance is the best way to receive this work. I hope that my writing encourages you to find out more and, in the meantime, is a helpful pointer to improving yourself somewhat in your current circumstances.

I also hope that this book can be used alongside a series of Alexander Technique lessons to help with the fuzziness surrounding the learning process at the beginning!

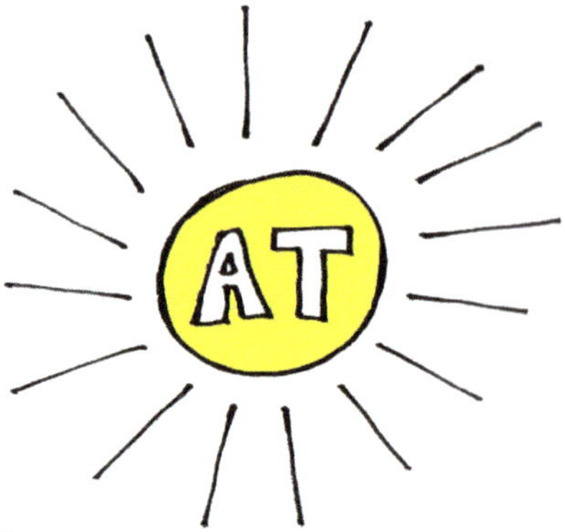

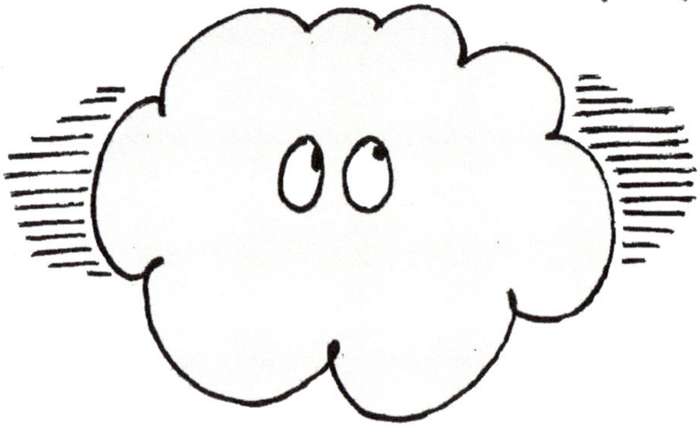

> Alexander established not only the beginnings of a far-reaching science of the apparently involuntary movements that we call reflexes, but a technique of correction and self control which forms a substantial addition to our very slender resources in personal education.
>
> **George Bernard Shaw –**
> **Writer, Nobel Prize Winner for Literature**

CHAPTER EIGHT

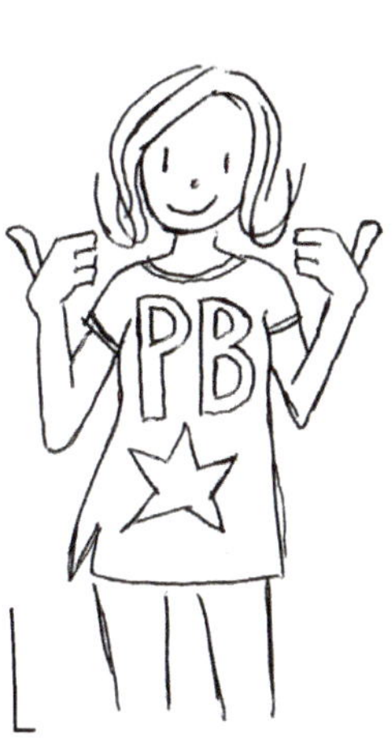

BE YOUR PERSONAL BEST AND MAKE YOUR BEST PERSONAL

Did you know that the Alexander Technique is an integral part of the curriculum at many top schools of performing arts around the world? These include **RADA**, **LAMDA**, the **Royal College of Music**, the **Royal Academy of Music**, the **Guildhall School** and the **Juilliard School**, to name but a few .

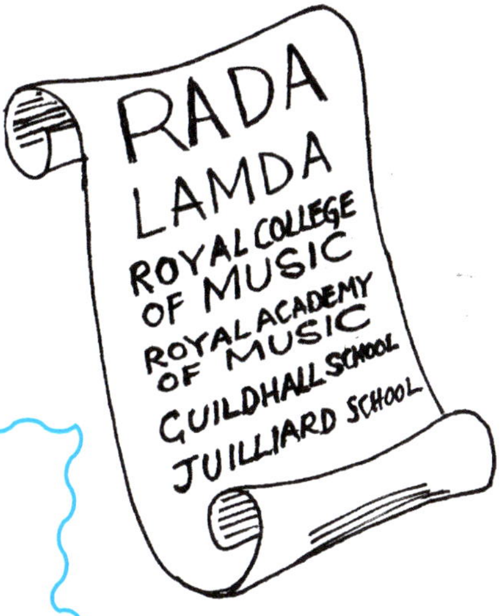

"the ALEXANDER TECHNIQUE can be SUSTAINING

it is something that if learned well, can be carried along with you for the REST of your LIFE . . .

IT GIVES YOU CONFIDENCE to be WHO YOU ARE when you are up in front of an audience . ."

Patrick Maddams –
Managing Director, Royal Academy of Music

Some prestigious public and private schools also have resident Alexander Technique teachers for their music scholars. Some also have AT as an extra-curricular activity for pupils to learn how to use their body well, to help with performances and to enable them to use their instruments efficiently, preventing or limiting the opportunity for physical injury.

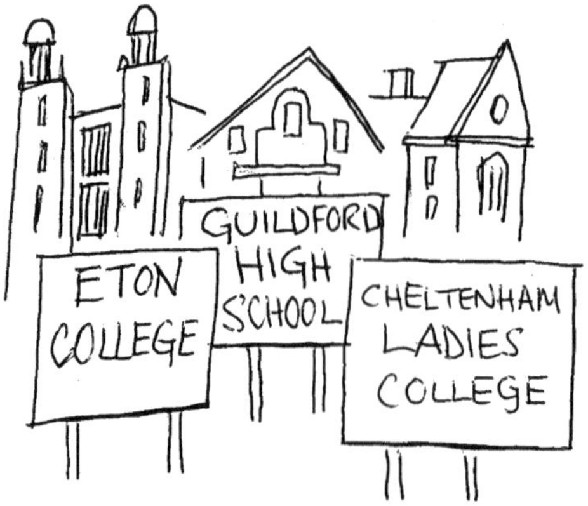

AT also teaches students the invaluable gift of presenting themselves in the best way. Positive body language with a resonant voice is a winning combination and an invisible advantage that will be of huge benefit. A few examples of such schools are: Eton College, Cheltenham Ladies College and Guildford High School .

Many forward-thinking companies are also employing Alexander Technique teachers to help their employees achieve health and wellbeing at work.

Happy, healthy people are, of course, productive. What a wise investment and how beneficial to be such a lucky employee!

This list is by no means exhaustive: Google, Disney, UBS, Merrill Lynch, Goldman Sachs, Victorinox, ICI, The Guardian, BBC, Chanel, City Lit, Hewlett-Packard and the British Library .

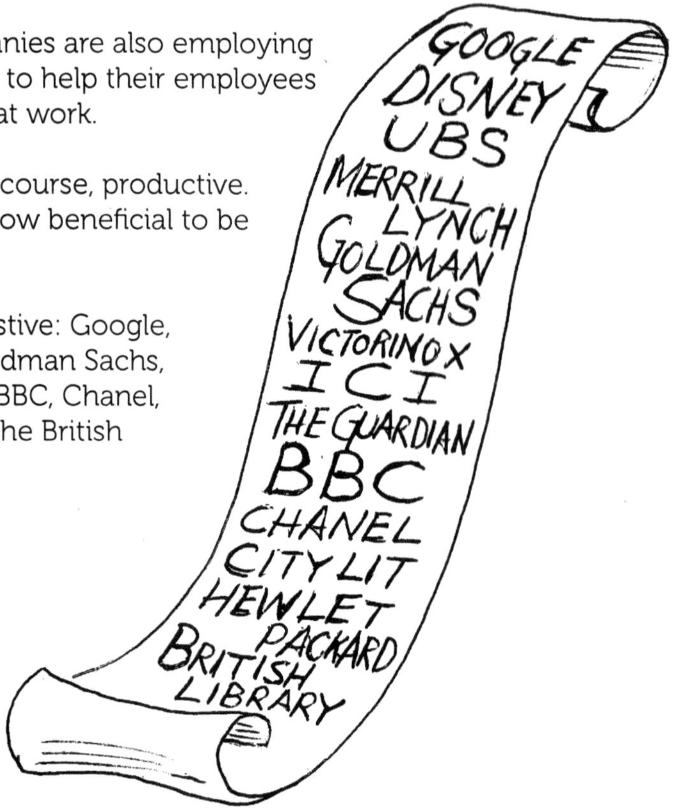

And if you're thinking to yourself, "But, I'm not a performer..." Oh but you are !

Everyone needs to be able to perform well in their own life. We are all playing the lead role in our own lives.

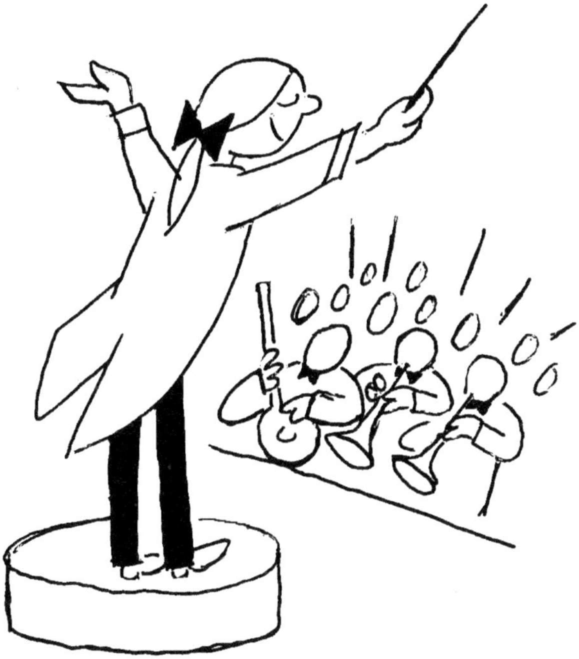

How would it be if we could express ourselves clearly and honestly? Communicate with ease? Allow differing opinions to be heard and respected? Be physically well and robust? Able to meet the challenges of a frenetic, demanding work and life, and retain a strong physical self to be able to participate fully in a fulfilling active, fun and social private life?

IT IS POSSIBLE!

HOW?

You can integrate AT principles into your own life and then you become the **BEST** version of you that is possible. Fulfil your own potential.

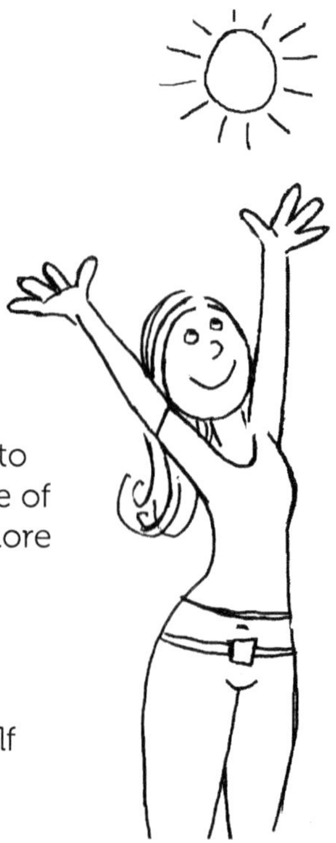

YES, THE SKY'S THE LIMIT !

Who knows what hidden talents lie beneath self-sabotage? Wouldn't you like to find out?

Life is not a rehearsal.

Understanding your body, knowing how it works, listening to it and respecting it pays huge dividends. This gives us peace of mind and makes all of our activities mindful. We become more **PRESENT**.

You've already noticed some physical habits that may have been limiting movement, or making it more difficult, if not causing you actual pain, by learning about your physical self earlier on in the book. What if you could consciously direct your thoughts, too, in the same way?

Guess what! **You can!**

You know we also have habits of thinking. They're not all entirely personal either. We have cultural thinking habits. Society shapes our thought patterns, too. And there are also family patterns and habits that come into our behaviour too .

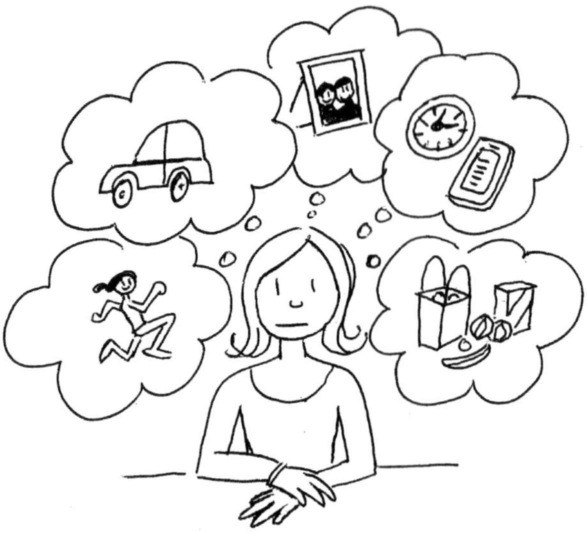

Now this is where the journey **REALLY** begins.

Many people think they've 'got' the Alexander Technique when their physical ailments have 'gone away'.

Oh no! This is only the **START** if you wish to explore yourself further and go deeper and find out **WHO YOU ARE!**

Who do you think you are?

I love the TV programme of the same name. I find fascinating the idea of discovering the secrets and lives of previous generations by going back into our personal history.

We **ALL** have a history. We are all a product of that familial line whether we like it or not. It is part of us .

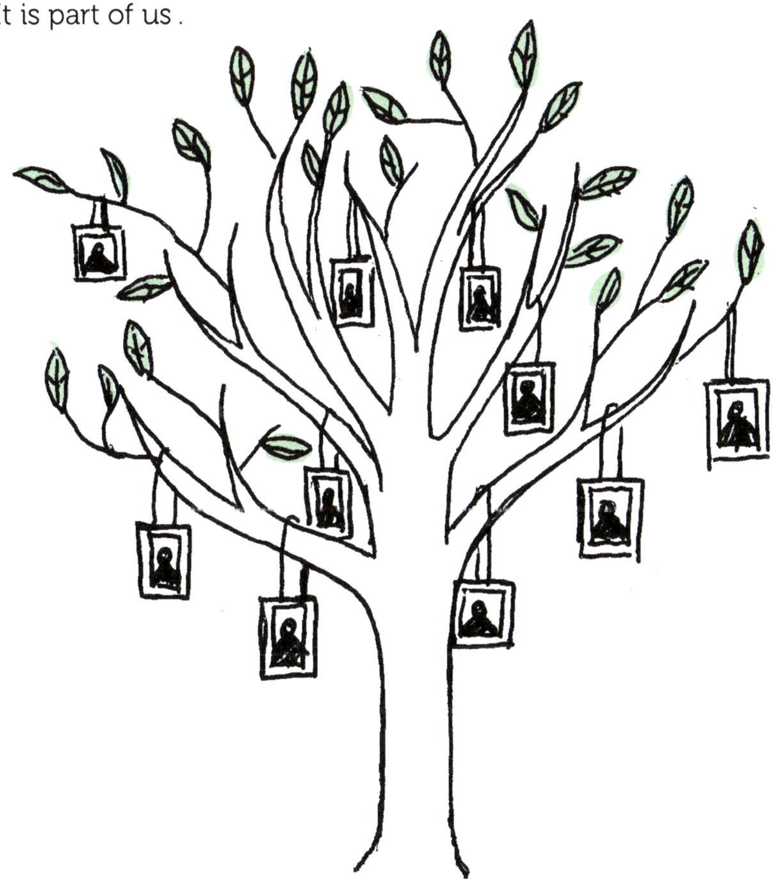

We **EMBODY** our history, our life experiences, our memories, thoughts, emotions and feelings. All of it is within.

SO if there are any issues, you'll find that they get 'stored' in the tissues!

Interesting? It's a fascinating journey when we begin to question

HOW we do things

WHY we do it that way

and... IS there a different way?

Explore. Experiment. Find out. It's amazing what you learn along the way .

It's sometimes painful (physically, emotionally, spiritually) but ultimately it's liberating to let go of what no longer serves you.

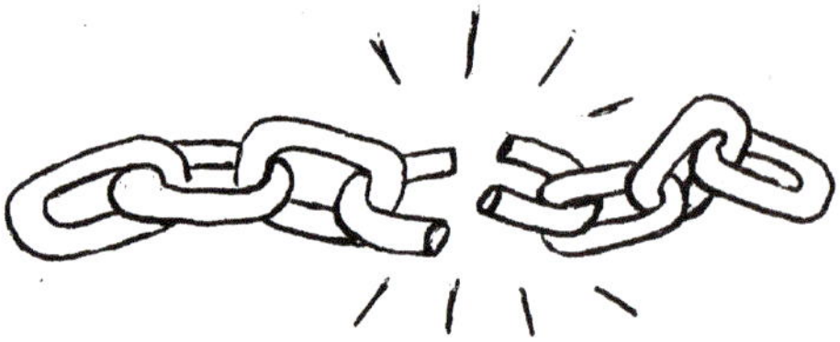

It frees **YOU** from the shackles of unnecessary tension and frees those around you, too. You also stop the unhelpful habits from continuing unconsciously further down the family line. Hurray!

Don't be daunted: the **FEAR** of exploring is inevitable, but what you should find is that by facing the unknown, the fear diminishes and the reality is usually more palatable than the imagination led us to believe.

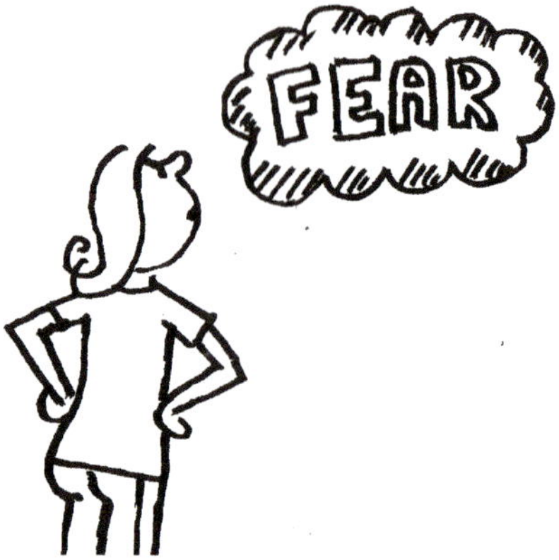

Confidence

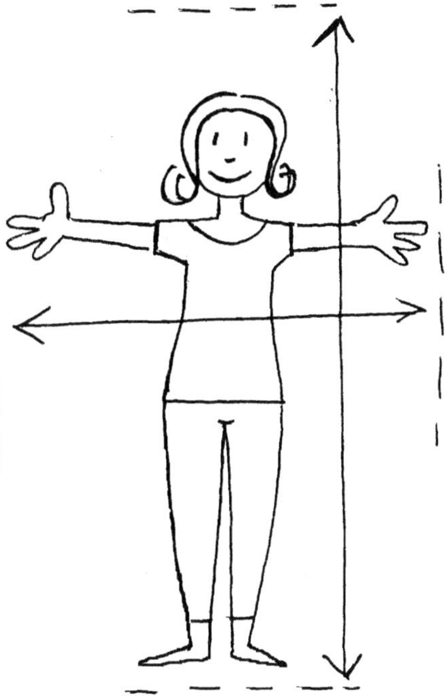

When you allow yourself to be something approaching your full height, your full width and depth, it's very liberating **PHYSICALLY** and **MENTALLY**.

You literally **FIND YOUR FEET**. And you also literally start being comfortable in your own skin.

Learn how to be authentically you **AGAIN**. We were all authentically ourselves when we were born.

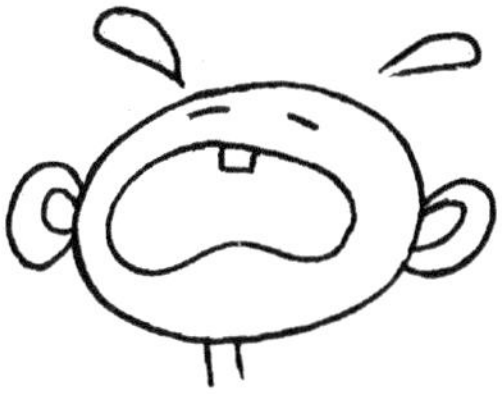

You don't hear of shy babies too quiet to ask for food, do you? No! Babies **DEMAND** food when they are hungry and are loud in their requests, too. So, you see, a lack of confidence is learned and adopted behaviour. Therefore, we can unlearn it and decide to subtract certain behaviour from ourselves that may be preventing our true nature from shining through.

To find your confidence again, learn how to use your body well again, adopt Alexander's principles into your life and your confidence will naturally start to return.

You can make yourself conscious of your habits so that anything **UNNATURAL** starts to become obvious and then you can choose it or not. **YOU** get to decide how you want your body and your self to behave.

All our life experiences become richer if we choose to engage with life fully by integrating ourselves and becoming congruent with our true nature. External circumstances can be seen as just that – external to ourselves. If we take care of our internal selves, some balance can be restored as to how we react and respond to those circumstances.

Performance

Being able to express oneself clearly is a gift that is everyone's birthright! Learning the Alexander Technique enables us to reconnect with our true feelings. Knowing how to 'get out of your own way' is liberating physically and allows our body language to reflect our thoughts and feelings truthfully. Thus, we present an honest version of ourselves to the world.

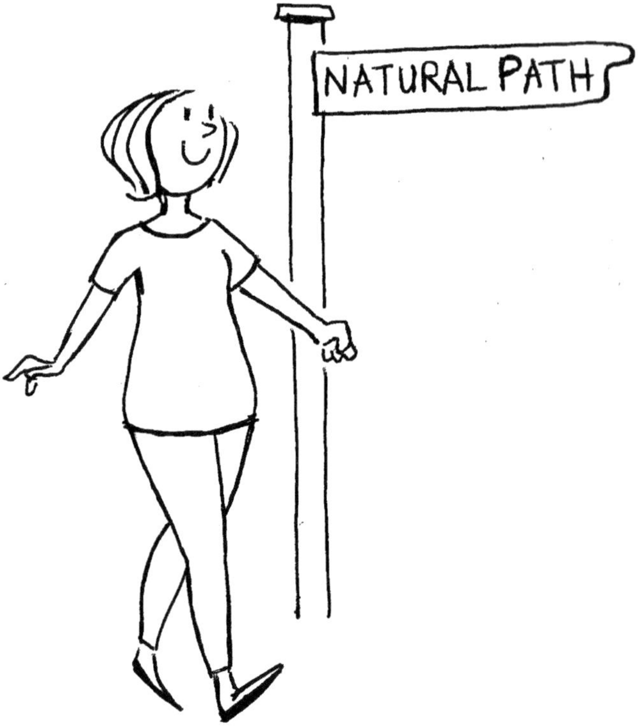

This makes things much less confusing for others. Like it or not, we all read body language. Its cues are understood immediately.

Once you learn the Alexander Technique you become more wholly congruous with your intentions and those are reflected honestly in your body.

You start getting 'wise' to others, too. Suddenly intuition and gut reactions can be heard, respected and listened to, keeping you closer to your natural path and less likely to fall prey to others. All the senses are more finely tuned, as well. Again, this is enormously helpful in 'reading' a situation. Forewarned is forearmed!

If you are an actor or musician, being able to perform on stage is a necessary requirement, as is the importance of expressing emotion and feelings accurately. That's what makes a 'good' performance: compelling, honest presence. So, again, we come back to clear, authentic body language.

It is ever more important in today's technological age to be aware of our actual thoughts and feelings. Too often now we are distracted by devices like computers, laptops and smart phones, and our attention is taken **OUT** of ourselves and into something external to us. Imbalance is common.

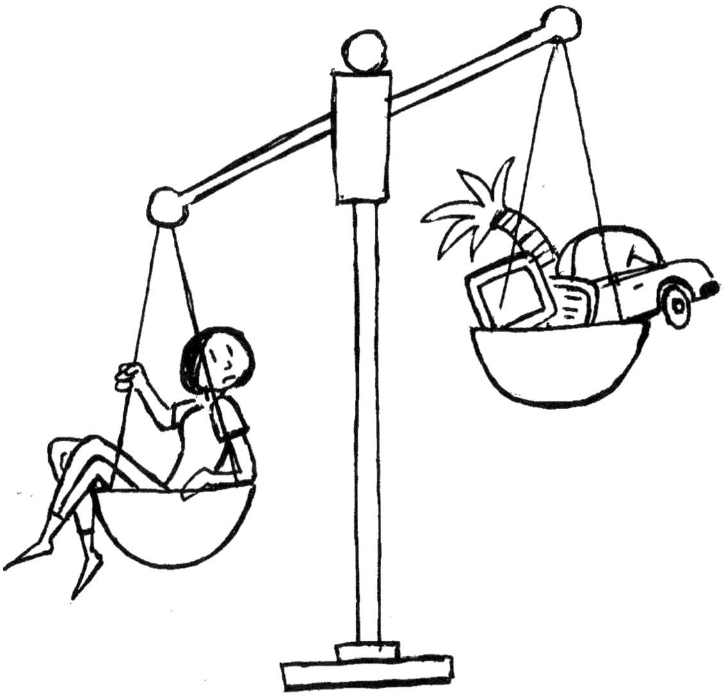

I stress the importance here of learning how to reconnect with ourselves and reality; to retain our best co-ordination and to remain physically active; and to be co-ordinated well during movement so that sedentary lifestyle problems no longer plague us.

We can rediscover our **CONNECTION** to life, to those around us, and to nature.

“

The Alexander Technique has been like magic and instrumental in getting me on the right path after a disc bulge in my lower back. I had become quite despondent and anxious at times due to a lack of improvement in my condition with conventional treatments, such as physiotherapy. One overriding feeling was fear at not getting back to a 'normal' state and I can honestly say that the Alexander Technique gave me the reassurance, positivity and tools to correct that. I am amazed at the multitude of ways in which my AT lessons have helped me, on both a physical and mental level. After a year of lessons I feel that I now have the tools and knowledge of how my body should work and, most of all, how I can help myself, wherever I may be.

Lisa Craig – Physiotherapist

”

CHAPTER NINE

HOW TO SIDE-STEP ANXIETY AND BEAT STRESS

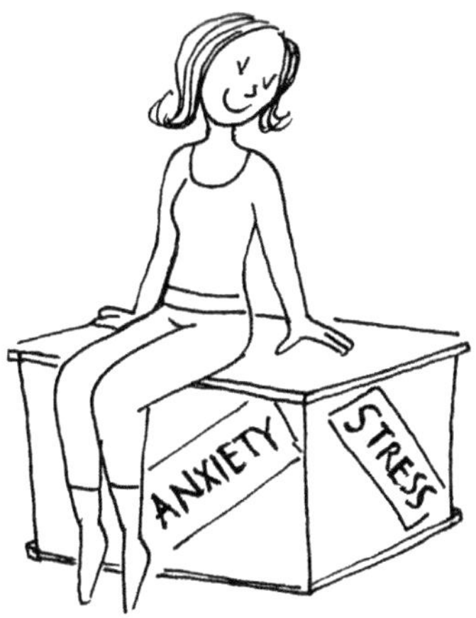

Modern lives are frenetic and the pace of living is fast, with many demands on us. We are time-poor and all of that stress is reflected in our posture. As a nation we are generally in poor physical shape. I'm noticing that, in fact, the younger generation are in worse shape than ever.

Our busy lives are here to stay – there's no going back. So, is there anything we can do?

Fortunately, there is. We can **CHANGE** our response to life. I touched on this in Chapter 7 but let's take it a little deeper.

The 'busy-ness' of modern life promotes stress and anxiety. That is very apparent in our bodies. So, by monitoring what our body is 'up to' we can manage to keep stress and anxiety at bay.

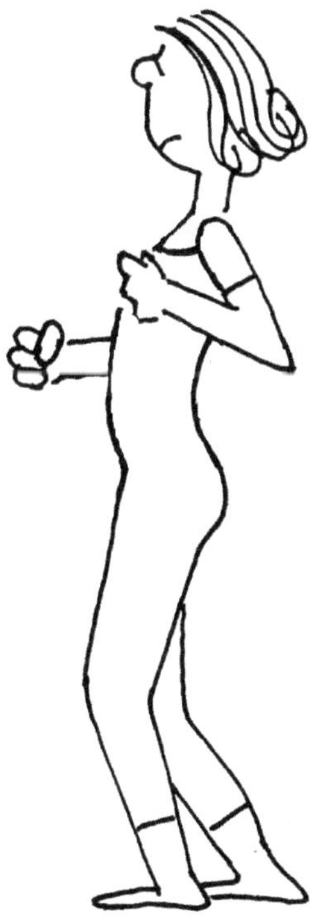

Let's look at what happens to us when we are experiencing stress and/or anxiety.

We tend to pull our heads back and down and we shorten and narrow in stature. We compress ourselves.

Why is that?

It's the survival mechanism being activated – the fight or flight response. It is our evolutionary gift and the best response for us in a life-threatening situation. It is the activation of the spring in our system that prepares us for the fight or a flight out of a dangerous situation.

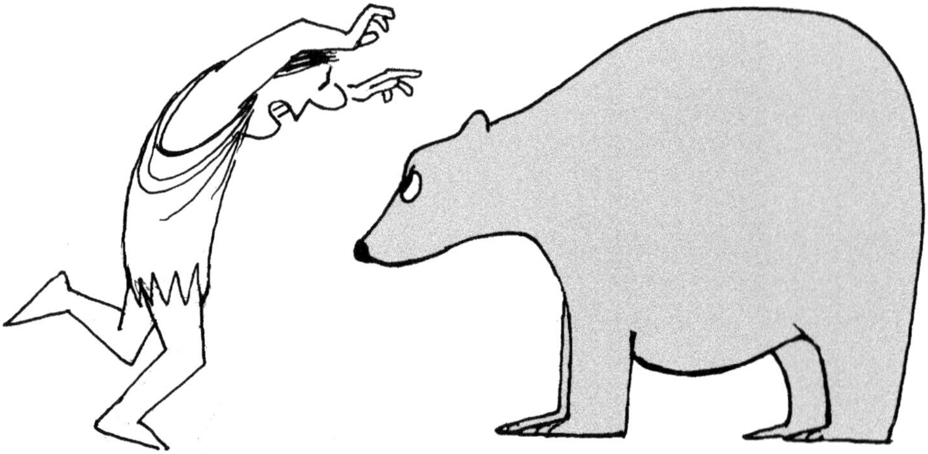

This response is no longer so relevant in modern times. Our stress is usually mental. We don't often have to run away or physically fight our way out of a dangerous situation. Rarely are we faced with an issue of survival.

In which case, our response to stress, to behave in a way in which our survival is threatened, is no longer appropriate for the majority of situations. We then 'hold' our compressed state unabated for long periods of time, which compromises our day-to-day functioning.

Our fight or flight response is activated frequently. Now we know about it and how it manifests in us, we can do something about it. Recognise it first and accept it is happening and then look at these suggestions of how to come out of it. Sometimes it could be viewed as an advantage in enhancing our senses, in which case these guidelines can also be helpful in riding the wave of extra energy deposited into the system via an adrenaline rush.

Coming out of an anxious, stressed state

How can you do this? By taking charge and making conscious your reaction to a situation. Ask your mind to quieten down its mental chatter. Pay undivided attention to yourself.

Find your feet. Ground yourself fully. Free all your natural hinges. Then send your AT directions:

- Ask your neck to free itself.
- Allow your head to move forwards and away from the top of the spine.
- Let your whole spine lengthen and whole back widen.
- Allow your knees to flow out from free hips, forwards and away.

Breathe!

Breathing

Shallow breathing is a factor of the flight or fight response. It's therefore commonplace in our everyday lives due to high levels of stress and anxiety.

There is a general level of unease and anxiety prevalent within many of us, and it increases as our modern lives fill up and get busier and more demanding.

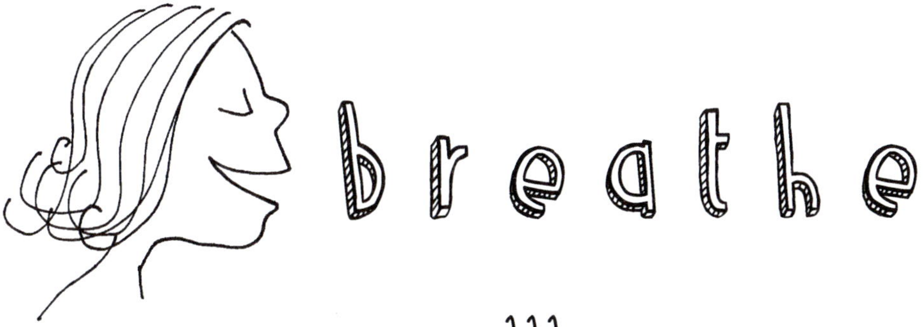

So, our attention to the breath should become even more important.
Many of us hold our breath when we're concentrating or listening! Check what you're doing and check often.

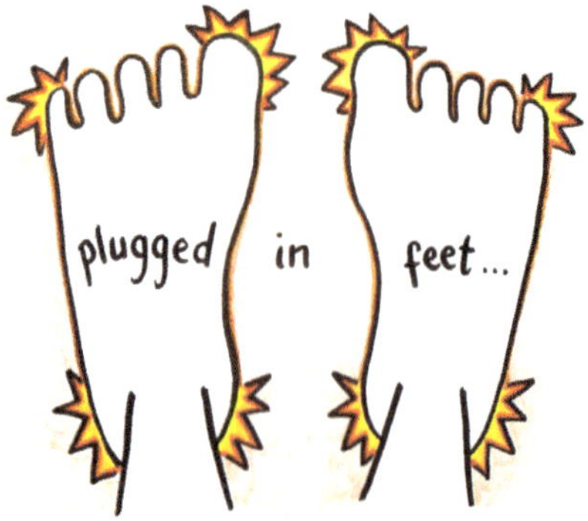

To break a cycle of anxiety ... **BLINK, BREATHE AND BE GROUNDED**. Here's a simple way to come out of an anxious state. I find this very easy to access, even in highly charged situations.

NOTICE if you're breathing ...if you're blinking ...
and if your feet are actually contacting the ground on these three points: the base of the big toe, the base of the little toe and the heel.

NOW ... breathe out gently, wherever you are in the cycle of respiration...as if you're blowing a feather across the room, until you have exhaled all the air in the lungs.

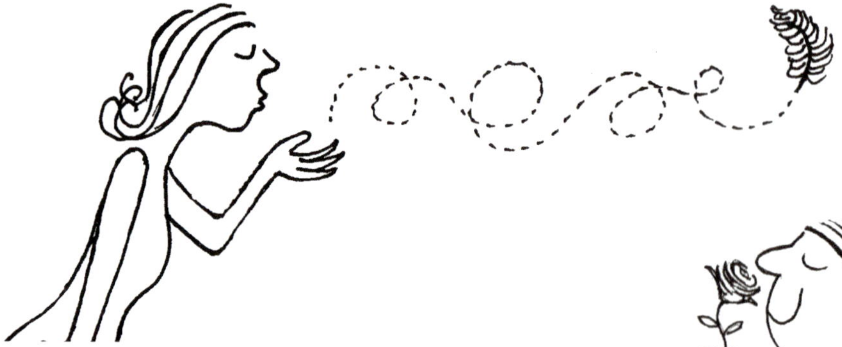

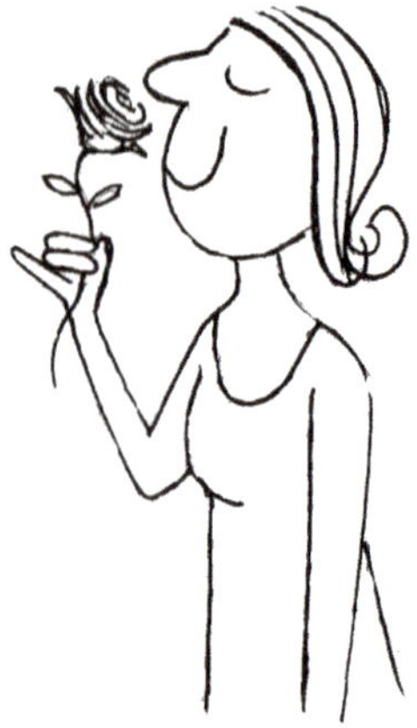

Now **STOP**, close your mouth, and wait quietly for the breath to come in **THROUGH** the nostrils and ... add in the thought that you are going to be smelling a delicious scent, something you **LOVE** to smell, such as a rose, freshly cut grass, the sea air – whatever **YOU** love – and do this twice more. This calms down the nervous system and allows your self back into the present moment.

Blink gently and softly, a few times slowly, and soften the gaze. Under stress we tend to stare and freeze the eyelids. Break this cycle and feel the stress melting away.

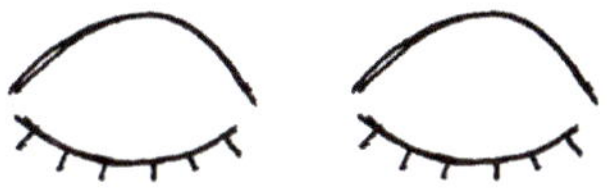

BE GROUNDED.

Our feet already want to run away when we're in the stressful moment; our muscles are already primed for this action ... **SO** bring your attention to your feet. **NOTICE** if they are actually making contact with the ground. How is your body weight distributed right now? Share your body weight evenly between both your feet. Allow the feet to fully accept the support of the floor. Let your toes lengthen away from your heels. Feet are springy in life – are yours? Let them receive the information the floor is offering. Now you have found your feet, land and re-evaluate your circumstances ...

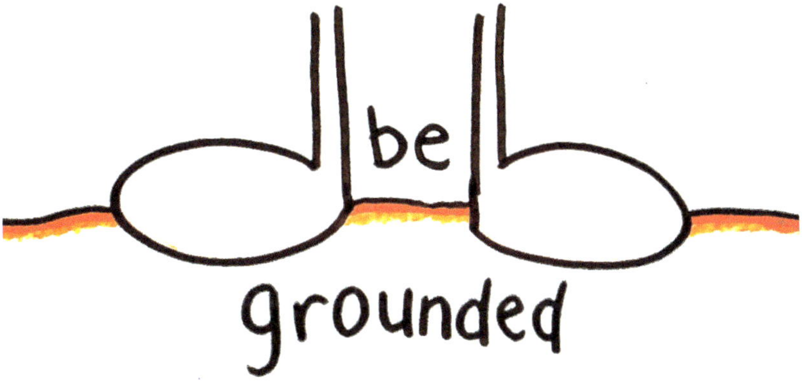

It's usually not that bad after all – it's just that our whole system had been compromised by the survival mechanism inappropriately being employed unconsciously by us. Awareness is the key – simply paying attention to your actual circumstances and bringing in those three helpful tips – blink, breathe and be grounded - allows the body to reorganise, and then awareness begins to expand again and the world looks like a friendlier place!

Enjoy!

The 'Whispered Ah'

This is one of Alexander's classic procedures. It is an extremely effective way of calming down from stress or anxiety. It's more involved than the previous exercise of blowing the feather/ smelling the rose but does give better results. As ever, I'm going to recommend most highly that you ask a qualified teacher to show you how to do this.

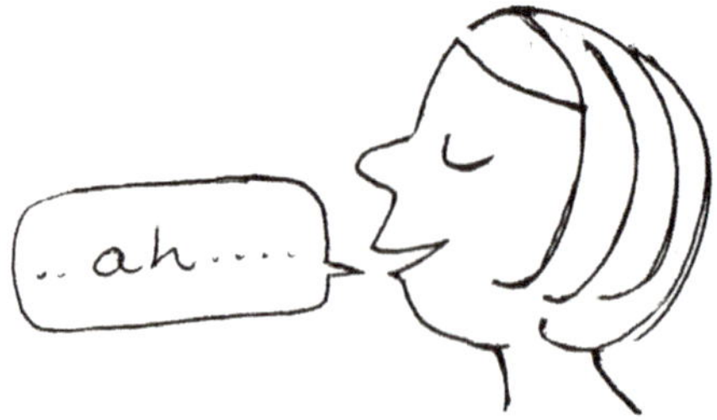

The 'Whispered Ah' is a vocal exercise that encourages openness in the neck, throat and around the vocal cords. It's a brilliant tool for those who use their voice professionally – singers, teachers, public speakers, for example – but, in fact, we can all benefit hugely as we all need to communicate well. Under stress, the throat constricts and our voices become very small!

I really hope these simple tips help you to manage nervousness, nip anxiety in the bud and manage stress better. Nothing replaces a hands-on AT lesson for deep understanding and the ability to help yourself under difficult circumstances.

Go on! Invest in yourself!

" I view my Alexander Technique sessions as 'meditation for the body'. The more stressed my life is at work and elsewhere, the more I feel I benefit from this oasis of calm, which is effectively an opportunity to 'restore to factory settings' by pressing a physical reset button.
It also tends to carry over into the rest of my life – I regularly stop at a local café for a cup of tea on my way home from an AT session and ruminate on the things that I've learned or realised during the session, and on the many broader implications that I could take from these into my life in general. And, every time, I come away with another little light bulb moment. Nothing big, nothing too momentous, just a genuinely useful thought for the week.

Janet Davis – Management Trainer, Dance Teacher and Ski Instructor "

CHAPTER TEN

FACING THE FUTURE

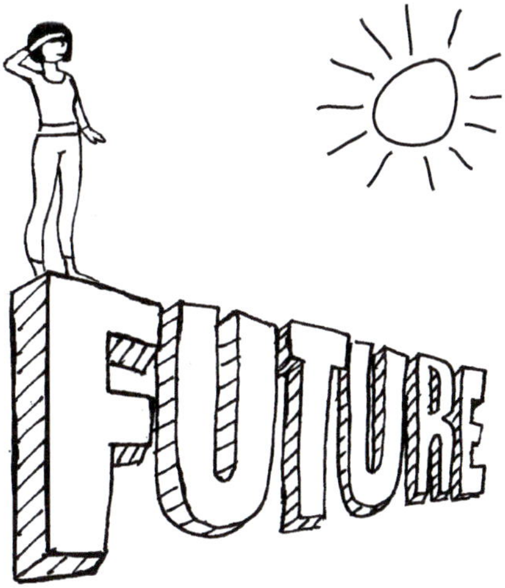

What next for you?

You now have some practical ways to improve your co-ordination at your disposal. You have a plan for life!

How does that feel?

You can embrace your future knowing how to be grounded and free of unnecessary tension. You have a method by which you can restore balance to your **WHOLE** self in order to respond appropriately to your ever-changing circumstances, whatever happens.

In short, I hope you now realise that the Alexander Technique gives you back **OPTIONS** and **CHOICES** .

So **YOU** are in control of you and your life again.
As if by magic!

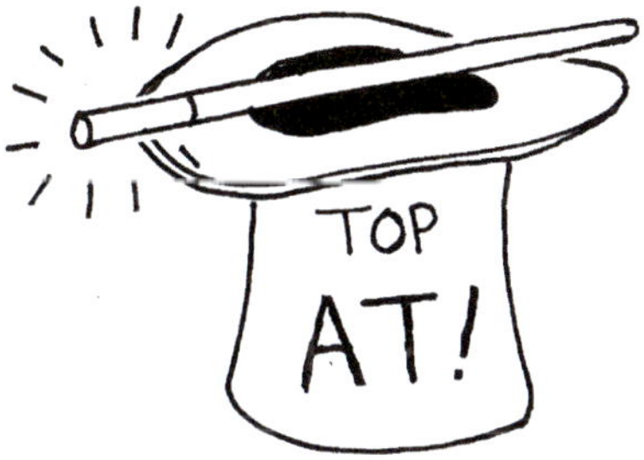

ABRACADABRA !

Moving more easily and freely is a possibility, as is being flexible and strong.

Using the four simple Alexander directions is the way to an open relationship with your body, offering you a strong connection to your natural true self.

Options for your Alexander Technique journey

To find a teacher, start by searching for someone local to you.

The Society of Teachers of the Alexander Technique **(www.stat.org.uk)** has a directory of teachers, as well as a list of affiliated societies overseas to aid your search if you live outside the UK.

A fantastic global resource is Robert Rickover's **www.alexandertechnique.com**, which offers a wealth of information within. You will find research, articles, videos, podcasts and much more here.

Do have a look at my website **(www.angelabradshaw.com)** for up-to-date news and blogs from me, or follow me on social media – I'd love to connect with you!

You may be interested in reading a study published by The British Medical Journal (bmj.com/content/337/bmj.a884) that demonstrated that 24 lessons in the Alexander Technique will reduce back pain by 86%. The total number of patients taking part in the research was 579. Of those, 144 took 24 lessons.

> Every man, woman and child holds the possibility of physical perfection; it rests with each of us to attain it by personal understanding and effort.
>
> **F. Matthias Alexander,**
> **Developer of the Alexander Technique**

Are you ready to lighten up?

My big vision for the Alexander Technique

I'd love to see a world where everyone :

- knows how to use their body well
- embodies their true nature and functions at their best
- has enhanced self-awareness and self-respect
- is empowered to be themselves

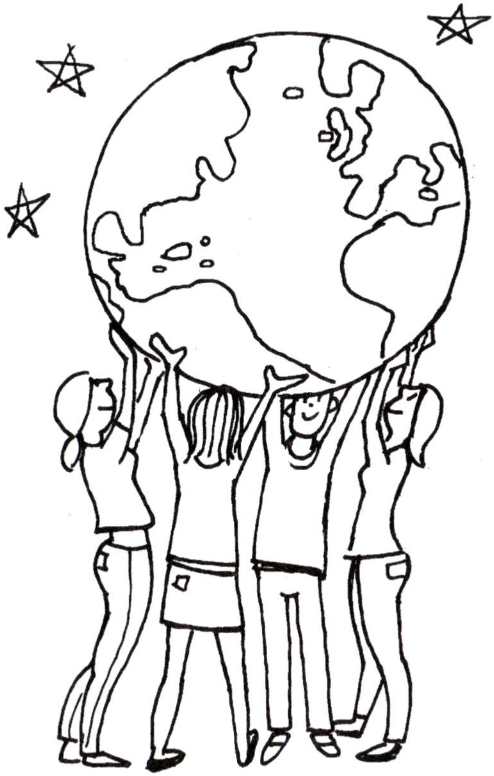

So

- Where are you now?
- How are you?
- Where are you going?
- What do you want?
- What are your expectations?

Send your directions ... breathe ... pause ... and move forwards freely and with ease.

Welcome your world, explore with curiosity and interest, and wholly engage with it .

Enjoy!

ACKNOWLEDGEMENTS

This book could not have happened without the inspiration, impetus and help from many people and I would like to **THANK YOU ALL** from the bottom of my heart.

In particular I would like to give huge thanks to Claire Holgate and Adrian Burrows for their amazing illustrations, and also to Ed Peppitt for holding my hand in my first foray into publishing.

Thanks too for the generosity of spirit afforded to me by Robert Rickover, Ron Colyer, Ilana Machover and Dr Miriam Wohl – my AT senior colleagues - for reading through my draft book, and lending advice.

There are so many others - it's impossible to name everyone who has helped me on this journey, but I want you all to know how much it's been appreciated.

Enormous special thanks too to my family for their unwavering love, support and help in this project. I feel lucky indeed